Death to
BULLYING

Death to
BULLYING

Dale Hirons
Robert Hirons
Gary Hirons

authorHOUSE®

AuthorHouse™ LLC
1663 Liberty Drive
Bloomington, IN 47403
www.authorhouse.com
Phone: 1-800-839-8640

Published by AuthorHouse   08/08/2013

ISBN: 978-1-4918-0182-6 (sc)
ISBN: 978-1-4918-0181-9 (e)

Library of Congress Control Number: 2013913858

Contents

Prologue

The purpose of this book is to inform students, parents, teachers and School Boards what steps they can take to stop bullying in our schools.

The first step is to understand that bullying cannot be allowed to take place. Bullying is to be considered an act of assault, is never justified, is never excused.

The second step is to understand that a bully is someone who feeds off the suffering and pain that they inflict on others. The bully looks for the most vulnerable child (usually those with special needs, as they are the easiest to victimize) and they enjoy every moment of their victim's melt-down. Only a true sadist would derive pleasure from harming an innocent child while encouraging others to enjoy the spectacle.

The third step is to realize that so-called experts have no vision of what a bully is. These people do more harm than good to the victims by continually offering programs to try to rehabilitate the bully, never realizing that they love to inflict pain.

We tend to think of bullying as boys using physical contact. Too many of us don't see the danger of girls using exclusion and isolation as a means of bullying and inflicting pain and suffering. This was just a prelude to the advent of the internet which now uses tools such as Facebook and blogs, and instant messages, knowing that the internet provider cannot be held responsible for what they post. Texting hurtful messages on phones is skyrocketing and, like the internet, there is no one who is willing to assume responsibility for monitoring what is being said.

What we are trying to do is to tell everyone that until they realize what a bully is, and what harm the bully is doing, our children will continue to be at the mercy of the animal that is destroying young lives. If you take the time to read this book, for the first time you may realize that you have in your grasp the necessary tools to protect a child before they look to suicide as the only way to put an end to this torment, as so many of our innocent children have. The victim must at all times be protected and the bully must at all times be held responsible—up to and including being charged with criminal assault.

We must work together if we want to stop bullying.

Facts about Bullying (2010)

Taken from www.bullyingstatistics.org

(There are about 160,000 children that miss school every day out of fear of being bullied.)

2.7 million students are being bullied each year;

One in seven students is a bully or a victim of bullying;

Revenge for bullying is one of the strongest motivations for school shootings;

56% of all students have witnessed bullying at school;

71% of students consider bullying as an ongoing problem

282,000 students are reportedly attacked in high schools each month.

Sources: makebeatsnotbeatdowns.org, olweus.org

Cyberbullying:

More than 50% of adolescents and teens have been bullied online;

More than 33% of young people have experienced cyberthreats online;

Over 25% have been bullied repeatedly through cell phones or internet;

Well over 50% do not tell their parents when cyberbullying occurs

Source: i-SAFE foundation.

Fewer than 20% of cyberbullying incidents are reported to police;

10% of adolescents have embarrassing or damaging pictures taken without permission by people using cell phones;

1 in 5 teens have sent or posted sexually suggestive photos of themselves to others.

Source: Hartford County Examiner

Cyberbullying victims are more likely are more likely to have low self-esteem and consider suicide.

Source: Cyberbullying Research Center.

We Have Serious Problems in Our Schools . . .

18% of children who worry about bullying said they wouldn't talk to their parents about it.

38% of disabled children worry about being bullied.

38% of young people have been affected by cyber-bullying.

41% of schoolchildren who are bullied online do not know the identity of the perpetrator.

41% of school staff witness at least one incident of bullying per week.

43% of the students fear harassment in the bathrooms at school.

46% of children have been bullied at school.

58% of students in grades 4-8 reported that they had mean or cruel things said to them online.

65% of lesbian, gay and bisexual young people have experienced homophobic bullying at school.

68% of teens agree that Cyberbullying is a serious problem with today's youth.

80% of Canadians feel that bullying is one of the biggest issues facing students today.

Sources: Statistics on Bullying; Stop Cyber Bullying; Bullying StaÂsÂcs; Research Canada

Governments are not doing enough

Parliament on Monday debated whether to study the need for a national anti-bullying strategy, based on a motion put forward more than six months ago by NDP MP Dany Morin. Morin urged kids who are bullied to speak up. "They should find a parent, a member of their family, a teacher or someone they trust . . . (to) make sure the bullying stops," he said.
Source: *Toronto Star*, Tuesday, October 16, 2012

Parents' Bill of Rights

- You have the right to have your child attend school safe from fear.

- You have the right to expect your school to have an effective anti-bullying program.

- You have the right to receive a copy of this program.

- You have the right to know what incidents constitute assault.

- You have the right to know what incidents constitute criminal assault.

- You have the right to know what incidents constitute school expulsion.

- If a bullying incident involving your child occurs, you have the right to be informed of the incident.

- You have the right to attend a meeting with the principal to discuss the details of the incident.

- You have the right to know the outcome of the incident.

- You have the right to know what steps will be taken to ensure the incident will never happen again.

- You have the right to ask for a report from the School Board if you receive no satisfaction from the teacher and/ or the principal.

- You have the right to seek legal advice if you have followed these steps and received no satisfactory answers from the school.

- You have the right to sue the School Board for gross negligence if neither the principal nor the teachers handled the bullying incident in such a manner that it will not recur.

Parents Support Group

Schools will need help from parents in their efforts to put an end to bullying in their school. The students need to know that we are all there for them.

Steps to forming a Parents Support Group

- Arrange a meeting of concerned parents.

- Organize a committee to oversee the meetings: chairman, secretary, treasurer, etc.

- Develop a set of goals for the group.

- Define your policies and procedures.

- Establish and maintain a specific start time for the meetings.

- Find a cordial meeting place.

- Prepare brochures with your aims and objectives to be given to prospective and/or new members.

- Have someone in charge of media exposure to promote the group's accomplishments and goals.

- Establish a fundraising committee to cover expenses. Challenge the group to come up with some creative and fun ideas.

- Develop an online communication system to correspond with each other.

- Organize related projects and activities for the group.

- Work with the Principal and the School Board in developing a safe environment for all students.

- Make sure all of the students' parents know about the support group and its accomplishments.

Warning to School Boards

The Supreme Court of Canada has ruled that schools do not do enough to protect children who attend classes. Some School Boards are now being sued by parents for gross negligence.

Programs that deal with expulsion, zero-tolerance, mediation and conflict resolution are proving to be ineffective, leaving School Boards open to civil action by parents. Personal injury lawyers are receiving calls from parents to represent them.

School Boards in Vancouver, Winnipeg, Ottawa, Waterloo and Owen Sound have bullying lawsuits ęled against them. The Bluewater District School Board in Owen Sound had four claims filed against it (totalling $34,000,000) for gross negligence. In a court case in Vancouver, the Supreme Court of Canada ruled that the School Board was liable because it did not do enough to protect a student. In incidents of bullying on school property—in which the bully and victim can be readily identified—the School Board can be held liable for not providing a safe environment for students.

Canadian Common Law has long held that the responsibility of School Boards, administrators, and teachers is "that of a reasonably careful or prudent parent. This includes the duty to protect students from any reasonably foreseeable risk of harm," (Roher 2007, p. 20)

Teachers and principals are placed in a position of trust that carries with it onerous responsibilities. When children attend school or school functions, it is they who must care for the children's safety and well-being. In order to teach, school officials must provide an atmosphere that encourages learning. During the school day they must also protect our children.

To a far greater degree than ever before, the Canadian judicial system is sending a strong message about bullying to School Boards that bullying is unacceptable, and as Roher notes "The Supreme Court of Canada has said that a threat is a tool of intimidation" which is designed to instill a sense of fear in its recipient.

In Toronto, at a conference hosted by The Canadian Association for the Practical Study of Law in Education, a paper was presented titled "Education's Perfect Storm" which advocated more lawsuits against schools. The paper said not to blame the bullies, instead hold someone responsible who has the resources to act and dampen bullying. That is the schools and the School Board.

Tips for the School Board

We have a program "Youth Behaviour Guidelines" that consists of an Anti-Bullying Policy that effectively deals with bullying in schools and contains information on preventing bullying.

This policy is very beneficial to School Boards as it effectively puts the onus on the bullies and includes law enforcement involvement. The policy is simple for the school to implement. Teachers will appreciate the fact that they are given the educational tools and also have the freedom to make changes they feel will be beneficial to the program.

This policy

- Expresses the need for an effective anti-bullying policy.

- Spells out what the various acts of bullying are.

- Tells which bullying acts constitute assault.

- Explains which bullying acts constitute criminal assault.

- Details when police should become involved.

- Helps determine when bullying acts should result in school expulsion.

Today many more parents are becoming aware of the fact that School Boards, if necessary, can be sued. Our program, if adhered to, can be a deterrent from being held responsible for gross negligence.

The Ontario Education Act states that:

- It is the duty of a teacher "to maintain under the direction of the principal proper order and discipline in the teacher's classroom and while on duty in the school and on school grounds."

- Therefore, if a teacher observes incidents of bullying, it is the teacher's duty to intervene.

- The principal's duty makes it incumbent upon him/her to prevent physical or mental harm to a student.

- The act states that it is a principal's duty "to maintain proper order and discipline in the school."

- The act makes it incumbent upon a principal to either suspend or expel a student whose bullying is inflicting *mental or physical harm* to another student.

- Section 161.1 defines the statutory duties of the School Board. It states that every School Board shall "promote student achievement and well being".

- Section 302(2) of the Act establishes that the School Board has the power to establish policies and guidelines with respect to disciplining children.

- A School Board may be held liable when it has not established guidelines to assist principals and teachers in disciplining bullies.

It is not our intention to encourage parents to sue School Boards. It is only their last resort. We want everyone to work together to give our children a good education without fear or hindrance from bullies. There is no place for them in our community and it is up to all of us to make them aware of the fact that we are fighting back.

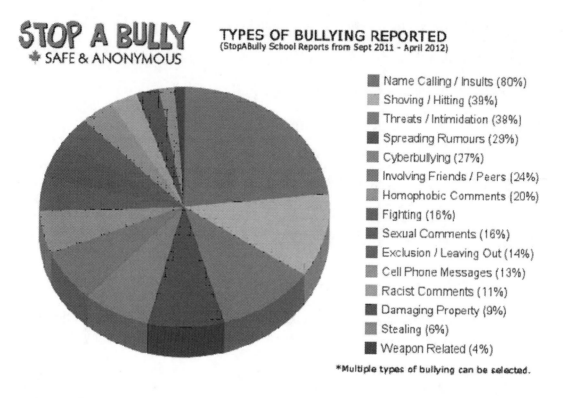

*Canadian Bullying Statistics; http://www.stopabully.ca/bullying-resources/bullying-statistics

Today's Youth Anti-Bullying Policy and Behaviour Guidelines

A program designed to educate today's youth, parents and teachers on how to end Bullying in our schools.

Introduction

To understand the best way to stop bullying, you should examine the tools that are in place to protect children from the act of bullying.

The United Nations Charter of Rights for Children states that:

- Every child has the right to an education;

- Every child has the right to be safe;

- Children who are physically, mentally or socially handicapped shall be given special treatment, education and care.

Canada signed on to this U.N. resolution thereby making the Federal Government responsible to protect children from bullying.

Not one so-called bullying expert can tell you what makes a person a bully so rather than wasting time reading what pseudo-experts have to say about stopping bullying,

Why not sit down and ask an expert.

The expert is the victim. For only he knows what the **FEAR FACTOR** is and is a true believer that this is what will be with him every day of his life.

The **FEAR FACTOR** is the fear of getting up every morning afraid to go to school, knowing that you will be the victim of physical bullying, social bullying and/or psychological bullying. Every school day they will face this and, unfortunately, there will be no one to turn to for help. Some of them will be physically or emotionally handicapped, some will have a different sexual orientation, and some will have a different ethnic background.

They will face the **FEAR FACTOR** and in some cases will ultimately break down and give up fighting. They then will turn to suicide as the inevitable escape from this continual torment.

The true expert knows that the effects of bullying lasts a lifetime and never goes away.

At no time is the victim or victims ever a part of the solution.

Action/Response:

1. Bullying occurs when force is used to inflict pain on a victim without their consent.

2. The root cause of bullying is the enjoyment of inflicting pain and torment.

3. Methods used to bully a victim: physical, psychological, verbal.

4. What is bullying? An act of assault.

5. How can bullying be stopped? Treat it for what it really is.

6. When bullying escalates to criminal assault, then it becomes a criminal offence.

7. When a criminal offence occurs, law enforcement takes control of the situation and criminal charges are laid.

Zero tolerance should be interpreted as disciplining a bully when they break the school's rules against bullying. It should not mean punishing a student for any and all physical contact. What if it was an accident during a game? What if the alleged lie was told to get someone in trouble?

Program Description

Today's Behaviour Guidelines has compiled a program for anyone involved in our schools, including the students, teachers, staff and parents. This program is divided into three sections.

The first section is our Safe-School Anti-Bullying Policy. This policy is designed to prevent school bullying, which is becoming more of an epidemic each year. It contains detailed information on bullying and a one-of-a-kind school policy that details how to rid schools of bullying—starting in grade 1—and fosters a safe school environment for all ages. The policy combines a strict approach with rules and punishment guidelines, school questionnaires used for needs assessments and evaluation, and classroom guidelines for every grade.

> **According to a national survey commissioned by Care.com Inc., bullying and cyberbullying have eclipsed kidnapping as the greatest fear that parents have regarding their child's safety. Source: www.abilitypath.org/areas-of-development**

The second section focuses on Autism Spectrum Disorder, the fastest growing development condition in the Western world. New light is continually being shed on this problem, and its impact on families, daily. All special needs children need special attention, and we have to become better informed so we can identify them, understand their unique condition, and help them.

The third section is an informative guideline focusing on many of the ever-evolving issues that today's youth face. It is designed to assist anyone involved with our children. The eight chapters discuss suicide, drugs, alcohol, tobacco, peer pressure, abuse, eating disorders and sexuality.

Part One

The Anti-Bullying Policy and Guidelines

Authors' Note: The Anti-Bullying Policy was endorsed by the Ontario Principals' Learning Foundation.

The Educational Program was awarded a grant from the Canadian Federal Government's National Crime Prevention Program.

An introduction to Bullying and
The Safe-School Anti-Bullying Policy

<u>Definition</u>

Bullying is never justified, nor is it excusable as kids being kids, just teasing, or any other unacceptable rationalization. Bullying should be seen as a relationship problem between two or more people, where one uses the assertion of power through aggression, physically or verbally, to cause a power differential between the bully or bullies and the victim. These actions can be repeated over long periods of time, or be short in duration.

Bullying is found worldwide and knows no economic or ethnic boundaries. Most children will be subject to one or more types of bullying at some point. The effects of being bullied range from low self-esteem, physical illness, anxiety, post-traumatic stress disorder, celibacy, and/or depression, which often leads to suicidal thoughts or actions. The effects on those who frequently witness bullying can be the feeling of powerlessness, fear, guilt, and empathy for the victims.

A school that doesn't properly deal with bullies creates a climate of fear, disrespect, lack of control and an environment that interferes with students' learning.

<u>Types of Bullying</u>

<u>Physical</u>

This is the use of an aggressive physical action to create an imbalance of power. Physical bullying tends to be swift and effective. It generally consists of pushing, hitting, tripping, punching, and any other unwanted physical contact.

<u>Racism/Intolerance</u>

The bully uses verbal or physical threats in which an individual's beliefs, race, religion or sexuality/homophobia is their weapon.

Cyberbullying

The use of electronic devices such as computers and cell phones used to inflict psychological and/or social bullying takes many shapes and can be found in texts, posts, blogs, emails, and other networking websites.

Tactics may include the sending of text messages or images with the intention of hurting or embarrassing an individual. It may be the repetitive sending of unwanted messages which may include inappropriate sexual remarks, racial remarks, threats, or false statements, created to harass or humiliate the individual.

The drastic increase in cyberbullying is in part because of the ease with which today's attacker can do irreparable emotional damage while remaining anonymous. Like traditional social and psychological bullying, cyberbullying occurs twice as often with girls as opposed to boys, both as victims and bullies.

Internet tools such as Facebook, instant messaging and text messaging make it easy for bullies to solicit help from others who may have had no involvement with the intended victim.

These bullies seek to:

- Intimidate

- Control

- Manipulate

- Put down

- Falsely discredit

- Humiliate

These actions are:

- Deliberate

- Repeated

- Hostile

- Embarrassing

This form of bullying has resulted in many cases of suicide as a means of escaping this brutality.

Cyberbullying, a new menace, has to be stopped

(The term cyberbullying is attributed to anti-bullying activist Bill Belsey.)

The reasons teens give for Cyberbullying are: to show off; to be mean; to embarrass someone; for fun and entertainment; because they deserved it; and, in the majority of instances, to get back at someone. At first glance, it doesn't seem worse than any other form of bullying. If that were true, why is Cyberbullying making headlines for causing people to kill themselves? Attacking someone anonymously is cowardly and shameful. To do it until they feel compelled to take their own lives is criminal.

Young children (some too young) text on their phones with school friends or go online to chat with others. They are too naïve to know who and what is out there.

There is no such thing as privacy. Sending someone a revealing photo has even come back to humiliate adults who should know better.

Until those in control of the sources of communication children are using today are forced to take responsibility for the abuse of their creations, someone has to teach and protect our schoolchildren.

If other children refuse to believe and/or spread hurtful messages and photos, the bullies will have to come out of the shadows and be known for who and what they are. Then they can and will be prosecuted. Then those who are crying for help and not being heard in time will have the support they need.

Fight Back

If your child has been the victim of bullying, the following steps should be taken:

- Report the incident to the teacher;

- Ask for a report from the principal;

- Ask the principal what steps he/she has taken;

- Ask for the results of the investigation into the incident;

- Ask the principal what steps were taken to ensure the incident will not be repeated.

If you are not satisfied with the results, contact the School Board. If the School Board is lax in their duties, you may want to seek legal consultation for gross negligence. That is your right as a parent.

A step in the right direction . . .

Death to Cyberbullying

Though cyberbullying may be a recent addition to the dictionary, (or just a new word in general), it is all too familiar to students, and even parents and teachers.

In today's connected world, a student's life occurs as much on the internet as off it. As described on Cyber Bullying.org, "the use of information and communication technologies to support deliberate, repeated, and hostile behaviour by an individual or group, that is intended to harm others," and "it has become a big problem."

As social media becomes more and more a part of our lives, so to increases the forums for cyberbullying. However a recent Supreme Court of Canada may just change the playing field. On Thursday, the SCC ruled in favor of a teenage girl from Halifax, victimized on Facebook, allowing her identity to remain anonymous; a significant ruling in the protection of a child's privacy rights.

According to the *Legal Examiner*, a fake Facebook account was set up as the victim, in which malicious posts were made. In an effort to bring a defamation lawsuit against the bully, the victim and her parents requested that Eastlink, the internet service provider, provide the bully's identity, as Facebook had taken down the profile and ordered the bully's internet providers address. The family also requested their identities be kept anonymous and the judge consented.

The *Halifax Chronicle Herald* and Global Television opposed the ruling and the case eventually made its way to the Supreme Court of Canada. Of the decision, Justice Abella wrote, "If we value the right of children to protect themselves from bullying, cyber or otherwise, if common sense and the evidence persuades us that young victims of sexualized bullying are particularly vulnerable to the harm of revictimization upon publication, and if we accept that the right to protection will disappear for most children without further protection of anonymity, we are compellingly drawn into the case allowing the victims anonymous legal pursuit of the identity of the cyberbully."

UNICEF Canada-Toronto, September 27, 2012, posted an article on the internet:

Today's Supreme Court decision is an important step in protecting children from cyberbullying. It ensures that they can feel safe to seek justice without fear of revictimization.

Today's decision underscores the shared commitment of government, the courts and other responsibility-holders to protect the best interests and rights of children who are pursuing justice when they are victimized, in this case involving cyberbullying or harassment," said Marv Bernstein, UNICEFF Canada's Chief Advocacy Advisor.

UNICEF Canada intervened in the case to assert that A.B's rights under the UN convention on the rights of children were not taken into account by the lower courts. Canada is a signatory to the Convention on the Rights of the Child, which grants children the rights to special protection in court processes in recognition of their vulnerability.

Homophobic Bullying

These victims face the highest risk of bullying due to the perception of being of a different sexual orientation (gay/lesbian) and not wanting to risk having this become known.

These victims face the following forms of attack:

Verbal:

- Name calling
- Rumours
- Gossip
- Threats
- Sexual comments
- Jokes

Social Exclusion:

- Isolation
- Embarrassment
- Humiliation
- Intimidation

Physical:

- Obscene gestures
- Hitting
- Kicking
- Shoving
- Sexual threats

Homophobic Bullying and the Law:

In 1998 the Supreme Court of Canada stated that someone cannot be discriminated against on the basis of their sexual orientation.

In 2004 the Government of Canada included sexual orientation in hate propaganda provisions within the Criminal Code.

A recent human rights decision indicates that all schools have a positive duty to address a school-wide culture of homophobia.

*www.bullyfreealberta.ca/honmophobic_bullying.htm

Psychological/Social

Girls tend to prefer psychological and social bullying. These types of bullies use gossip or group exclusion, combined with verbal abuse, and their attacks are more difficult to spot compared to physical bullying.

Sexual

This type of bullying can include the initiation of unwanted physical contact or verbal contact that uses demeaning sexual remarks. This type of bullying is often found in connection with cyberbullying.

Special Needs Bullying

Autism Spectrum Disorder is the result of a problem that occurs during pregnancy when a malfunction occurs during the complex development of the brain, resulting in children born with sensory problems such as noise causing pain and panic attacks.

These children will have difficulty in school as their brain will pick up every noise in the classroom and cannot differentiate the teacher's voice from other noises.

Having difficulty forming friendships will make them the favorite target of bullies whose torment won't cease until the victim has a melt-down.

Types of Special Needs Bullying

- Physical: Hitting / Shoving / Tripping
- Psychological: Exclusion / Intimidation / Ignoring
- Verbal: Taunts / Slurs

Fact:

- More children are diagnosed yearly with autism than with cancer.
- Autism affects more than 2,000,000 children in the U.S. and Canada.
- Autism has no cure.

Verbal

When they use demeaning words to threaten others, these bullies often incorporate other specific types of bullying—psychological, racism or sexual.

Forms of bullying

Physical

- Hitting
- Kicking
- Punching
- Shoving

Psychological

- Verbal
- Insults
- Slurs

- Sexual harassment

- Racial comments

- Threats

Social

- Gossiping

- Rumours

- Ignoring

- Excluding

Direct vs Indirect

Direct bullying is the obvious physical or verbal attack where the bully initiates the contact face-to-face.

Indirect bullying is less obvious, the bully either uses someone else to relay the verbal or physical attack, uses exclusion, or the spreading of rumours.

In the last decade the wide use of cell phones and social networking websites has made cyberbullying very effective.

Bullying/Assault

At what point does verbal and physical bullying become assault? And when does it become **criminal** assault?

Assault occurs when physical force is intentionally applied to another person without consent, or by the act of threatening the use of force upon another individual.

Bullying can escalate to a criminal offence during physical bullying, verbal insults/ threats, harassment, intimidation, extortion and derogatory slurs which make a person fear for their safety.

Any student who has committed an act of assault in school should be subject to a criminal offence charge.

Criminal Assault

When bullying escalates to the point where it causes another person to fear for their safety, then that bully has committed assault, which should result in police intervention. At this time, the bully can be charged with a criminal offence.

When bullying becomes a criminal offence

- Assault

- Extortion

- Harassment

- Threats

- Intimidation

School Expulsion

After notifying the police, it should be mandatory for the school to expel a student if that student has committed any of the following acts on school property or in a school—related activity:

- Bullying (once our programme is implemented)

- Possessing a weapon;

- Using a weapon or threatening to use one to commit bodily harm to another person;

- Committing a sexual assault;

- Trafficking in illegal drugs or weapons;

- Committing a robbery;

- Giving alcohol to a minor.

The Final Step

If a student is expelled for bullying, our zero tolerance policy takes effect. This means that the bully must find another school to attend, or they have to be homeschooled. The victim must be made to feel safe and this cannot take place if the bully is allowed to return to the same school.

Bullies have to assert their power. That is more important to them than getting an education. If they lose control of their victim, they will need to exert more force to reestablish their superiority. They have to know who is in control, and that has to be the school staff. And the school staff will need the support of the parents and the police.

Statement of Intent

This school is committed to providing a policy against bullying and a place for our pupils to learn and grow safe from fear. We do not tolerate any form of bullying at our school. If an act of bullying does occur, it will be addressed quickly and effectively. We expect anyone who witnesses an incident of bullying to report the act to a staff member, under the promise of full confidentiality.

Safe-School Anti-Bullying Policy

Introduction

The Safe-School Anti-Bullying Policy is designed to prevent bullying from occurring at your school. It will educate students, staff and parents. The anti-bullying program focuses on the education of teachers and students along with swift consequences if an act of bullying takes place. It is easy to implement and can be modified to fit any educational environment.

Most bullying programs are "reactive" and deal with conflict resolution. These reactive approaches have included post-incident treatment for the bully, conflict resolution programs, student expulsion, or even nothing at all.

Unfortunately, bullies feel the need to torment others, and this policy will enable schools to learn how to develop safe environments for the students to learn without the fear of bullying. This policy is "preventative" and requires a school-wide effort that focuses on changing the behaviour of the students from day one, as well as the way teachers, faculty and parents deal with bullying.

Methods of Prevention and Education

1. The school will post a set of rules and the consequences, if an act of bullying occurs.

2. It will supply all students, teachers, staff and parents with copies of their anti-bullying policy.

3. They will emphasize the importance of reporting bullying incidents and how these actions make the school safer for everyone.

4. During the first week of school, the principal will conduct a seminar to introduce the policy and have a law enforcement official detail what constitutes criminal assault and its consequences.

5. The school will display a large poster in the school declaring that the school does not tolerate any form of bullying.

Anti-Bullying Rules:

1. There will be NO form of bullying tolerated at this school.

2. Any witness to an act of bullying is required to immediately report the incident.

For Grades 1-3 the Results of a Bullying Act are:

- First offence will result in the teacher explaining what act of bullying has occurred and that it is not allowed.

- Second offence will result in a meeting with the principal to discuss the incident.

- Third offence will result in the offender's parents meeting with the teacher, principal and guidance counselor to reiterate the rules of bullying and the discipline enforced if an act of bullying occurs again.

- Fourth offence will result in a meeting with a police officer to discuss the punishment (with emphasis on expulsion) for bullying.

For Grades 4-6 the Results of a Bullying Act are:

- First offence will result in a meeting with the school principal to explain the incident. The student will perform 4 hours of school volunteer work chosen by the principal (i.e. help clean school, help administration, etc.). The student will be reminded of the zero-tolerance policy (expulsion) and what repeat offenders will be subjected to.

- The second offence will result in a meeting with the student, parents, teacher, counselor and police representative. They will be told that there is no third chance and if detention doesn't put an end to this, expulsion is the school's next step.

For Grades 7 + the Results of Bullying are:

- The senior students are now subject to the full extent of the Safe-School Anti-Bullying Policy at a zero-tolerance school. Anyone caught bullying will be subject to either criminal assault charges or school expulsion. There is no second chance for these teenagers.

Needs Assessment

A needs assessment will help the school decide what areas have to be concentrated on. A comprehensive needs assessment should involve students, teachers, staff and parents. A staff and student survey should be done at the beginning of the school year to determine each student's knowledge of bullying and provide necessary information on the anti-bullying policy. The most helpful points will be simple and yet provide detailed information.

Some examples:

Is there a lot of bullying in your school?—Y / N

Do students get teased at your school in mean ways—Y / N

Are staff at your school helpful at stopping bullying—Y / N Do students try to stop bullying—Y / N

Do you know how to stop bullying—Y / N

What grade would you give your school for stopping bullying—A B C D F

A similar survey should be created to assess the knowledge of the student's parents. The survey should include a copy of the school's anti-bullying policy and must be signed and returned during the first month of school.

The school should collect data referring to past bullying incidents to enable them to assess the specific needs of the school.

The school's staff should assist in making changes they think are necessary to the survey, depending on the situations they feel need the most attention.

The staff should set goals that they feel are attainable for their school. Setting these goals will help the staff design and maintain proper discipline. Keeping statistics of bullying incidents and comparing them to the goals set by the school will let the staff know what areas need more attention and if their goals are being met.

Classroom Guidelines Grades 1-8

The Purpose of these Lessons

This grade-by-grade lesson guideline is a tool to teach the students what the various acts of bullying are and how it affects everyone at their school. The fact that everyone is participating reinforces the school's approach to the problem: awareness of all aspects of bullying makes it easier to eliminate it from the school environment.

Visual Aids

1. **Posters:** By using posters the students can see various acts of bullying and how it affects the victim.

2. **Quizzes:** At the beginning of the session there will be a quiz to determine how much the students know about bullying. At the end of the session there will be a quiz to determine how much the students have learned about bullying. This will enable the teacher to evaluate the program and to make any changes that they deem necessary.

3. **Role-Playing:** The students re-enact various scenarios of acts of bullying to show the pain it causes.

4. **Research Projects:** The students will be given bullying projects to do research on, so they can better understand causes and effects.

Class Time

Class time for grades 1-4 will be 30 minutes or less, due to the attention span of younger students. The teacher will determine how much time to devote to the lessons. Class time for students in grades 5-8 should be increased to 45 minutes.

Grades 1-2

Goals

Help the students understand:

- How proper behaviour in class leads to a happy and safe classroom;

- The definition of bullying and how it affects friendships;

- How to ask for help, who to ask, and how to help others;

- How to express themselves and be proud of themselves;

- How wrong bullying is and that bullies get themselves in trouble.

Lesson 1

Quiz

Materials Required:

Paper/pencils

The teacher will write on the blackboard that bullying will not be tolerated at this school.

- The teacher will explain to the students that bullying is hurtful and that it is not right to hurt another student.

- The teacher will arrange the students into groups of four.

- The teacher will ask each group to make a list of various acts of bullying.

Lesson 2

Poster

Materials Required:

Paper/Paint

- Teacher will explain to the class what bullying is.

- The teacher will arrange the students into groups of four.

- The teacher will have each group paint a picture of an act of bullying.

- The teacher will place the pictures on the wall and will have each relevant group explain that act of bullying

Lesson 3

Role-Playing

- The teacher will arrange the students into groups of four.

- The teacher will select incidents of bullying and have each group act out a scenario in which they perform one of them.

- The teacher will then explain what the act was and the effect that it has on the victim.

Lesson 4

Quiz

Materials Required:

Paper/Pencils

- The teacher will conduct a quiz to list the various acts of bullying.

- The teacher will then explain what the acts were.

- The teacher will thank all the students for doing so well and tell them that without bullying, the classroom will be a happy place to learn in.

The teacher will compare the results of the first quiz to the results of the second quiz to determine how effective the lessons were. If necessary, the teacher may make any changes deemed necessary to improve the program.

Grades 3-4

Goal
Help the Students Understand:

- How to identify bullying and how it affects others, while introducing a zero—tolerance approach.

- When, how and where to get help, if needed.

- How they can work together to create a bully-free environment. Have them discuss what qualities they believe they can use to create this.

Lesson 1

The teacher will write on the blackboard that no form of bullying will be tolerated at this school.

Quiz

Materials Required:

Pencils/Paper

- The teacher will explain to the class that bullying can generally be deemed as the use of aggression, intimidation, and/or cruelty with the deliberate intent to hurt the victim, whether it is physical or emotional.

- The teacher will assign a quiz to the students, asking them to write a list of what the various acts of bullying are.

- The teacher will keep the results of the quiz and compare these results with a quiz to be assigned as the final test.

Lesson 2

Role-Playing

The teacher will write on the blackboard: Direct Bullying is Physical: **Hitting, Kicking, Shoving.**

- The teacher will arrange the class into groups of four and will ask each group to perform a scenario on the action of a bully and the result of the act on the victim.

The teacher will write on the blackboard: Verbal Bullying is Taunting, Teasing, and/or **Racial Slurs.**

- The teacher will arrange the class into groups of four and will ask each group to perform a scenario on one of the above and describe the result of the act.

Lesson 3

Posters

Materials Required:

Posters/paint

- The teacher will arrange the students into groups of four and assign an act of bullying that they are to paint a picture of.

- The teacher will put one poster at a time on the wall and have each relevant group explain this act and how it would affect the victim.

Lesson 4

Role-Playing

The teacher will write on the blackboard the following types of bullying:

Indirect Bullying—Physical: Getting another person to commit an act of assault on someone.

Verbal: Spreading malicious rumours about another person.

Non-Verbal: Deliberate exclusion from a group or an activity, cyber bullying.

- The teacher will arrange the class into groups of four and assign each group a scenario relevant to one of these acts.

- The teacher will then ask the group to explain the act and its consequences.

Lesson 5

Poster

Materials Required:

Paper/Paint

- The teacher will arrange the class into groups of four and will assign each group an act of bullying to paint a picture of.

- The teacher will put one poster at a time on the wall and have each relevant group explain the act and how it affects the victim.

Lesson 6

Quiz

Materials Required:

Paper/pencils

The teacher will assign a quiz to list:

- What are different acts of Verbal Bullying.

- What are different acts of Non-Verbal Bullying.

The teacher will compare the results of the first quiz to the results of the second quiz to determine how effective the lessons were. If needed, the teacher may make any changes deemed necessary to improve the program.

Grades 5-6

Lesson 1

The teacher will write on the blackboard that bullying will not be tolerated at this school.

- The teacher will explain to the students that bullying is defined as the use of aggression, intimidation, and/or cruelty with the deliberate intent to hurt the victim, whether it is done physically or emotionally.

Quiz

Materials Required:

Paper/pencils

The teacher will assign a quiz to list the acts of:

- Direct Bullying.

- Indirect Bullying.

- Cyber Bullying.

The teacher will hand out the results of the quiz and will write the answers on the blackboard.

Lesson 2

Role-Playing

The teacher will arrange the class into groups of four and will assign a particular act for each group to show the bullying act and the effect on the victim.

Lesson 3

Internet

The teacher will assign each student the task of researching information on the internet and then preparing a report on:

- Cyber Bullying.

- The Short-term Effect on the Victim.

- The Effect on Others.

Lesson 4

Role-Playing

- The teacher will arrange the class into groups of four and will assign each group the task of acting out the results detailed in one of the reports.

- The teacher will ask the group to discuss the act and the results of the act.

Lesson 5

Posters

Material required:

Posters/paint

- The teacher will arrange the class into groups of four and will assign each group the task of painting a picture of Cyber Bullying.

- The teacher will put one poster at a time on the wall and have each relevant group explain what it means.

Lesson 6

Quiz

Materials Required:

Paper/pencils

The teacher will assign a quiz to list the acts of:

- Direct Bullying

- Indirect Bullying.

- Cyber Bullying.

The teacher will compare the results of the first quiz to the results of the second quiz to determine how effective the lessons were. If necessary, the teacher may make whatever changes deemed appropriate to improve the program.

Grades 7-8

These senior students should take part in the Anti-Bullying Policy by helping the younger students from the very beginning of the school year. When the junior students see how the older students act, it reinforces the program the teachers are developing and gives the young students visual evidence of how the policy works.

Goals:

- Reiterate the definition of bullying and its effects on others.

- Teach the students the strategies used to put an end to it.

- Teach them how to identify and deal with personal differences, and why it's wrong to stereotype.

- Teach them how to positively critique their own behaviour and how they can change for the better.

- Establish the bully-free classroom and continue this policy outside the school environment.

Lesson 1

The teacher will write on the blackboard that no form of bullying will be tolerated at this school.

Quiz

Materials Required:

Paper/pencils

- The teacher will explain to the class that bullying can generally be deemed as the use of aggression, intimidation and/or cruelty with the deliberate intent of hurting another person verbally, physically or emotionally.

- The teacher will assign a quiz to list the acts of Physical Bullying, Psychological Bullying and Social Bullying.

Lesson 2

Role-Playing

- The teacher will arrange the class into groups of four and will assign each group a particular act of bullying and to show the effect on the victim.

- The group will explain how they would feel if this act were committed on them.

Lesson 3

Internet

The teacher will arrange the class into groups of four and assign a group to do research and report on one of the following:

- Cyberbullying.

- Statistics on Teen Suicides Caused by Bullying.

- Effects of Homophobia on Teens.

- Bullying Statistics in Schools.

The teacher will ask each group to read out the results of the research project and to give their opinion of the results.

The teacher will then have these projects put into the school's monthly newsletter and give a copy to the Parents Support Group.

Lesson 4

Quiz

Materials Required:

Paper/pencils

The teacher will assign a quiz to list at what point does verbal and/or physical bullying become assault and at what point does it become illegal.

Answers:

- Assault occurs two ways. First, it is an assault for you to intentionally apply force to another person, directly or indirectly, when they do not consent to that force.

- Secondly, it is an assault for you to attempt, or to threaten by act or gesture, to apply force to another person, and that that person believes on reasonable grounds that you have the ability to apply that force.

Lesson 5

Quiz

Materials Required:

Paper/pencils

The teacher will review the results of the quiz and will write the answers on the blackboard.

The teacher will explain to the students that the following bullying acts constitute a criminal offence, and that is when the police become involved:

- Assault;

- Extortion;

- Harassment;

- Threats;

- Intimidation.

The teacher will assign a quiz on what student infractions warrant mandatory school expulsion:

Answers:

- Possessing a weapon.

- Using a weapon to cause or to threaten bodily harm.

- Committing physical assault on another person that causes bodily harm.

- Committing sexual assault.

- Committing a robbery.

- Giving alcohol to a minor.

Lesson 6

Quiz

Materials Required:

Paper/pencils

The teacher will assign the students a quiz to list the acts of:

- Physical Bullying.

- Psychological Bullying.

- Social Bullying.

The teacher will compare the results of the first quiz to the results of the second quiz to determine how effective the lessons were.

The teacher may make changes if deemed necessary to improve the program.

Children with special needs are more likely than those without special needs to be bullied on the way to school.

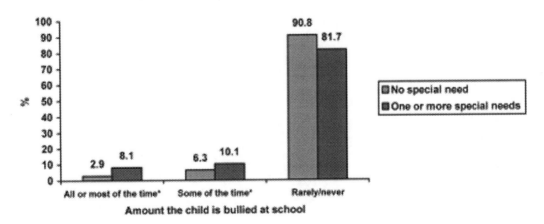

Figure 12
Distribution of children aged 10 and 11 with and without special needs, by how much they are bullied at school, 1994

*Canadian Council on Social Development, *Children and Youth with Special Needs*, page 30.

Part Two

Autism Spectrum Disorder

Chapter One

The Story of Autism

Autism Spectrum Disorder (ASD) is the fastest growing development condition in the Western world. Fifty years ago, it was considered rare, affecting one in every 10,000 children. In 2006 the estimate was one in every 110, today it is one in every 88—an increase of nearly 25 percent—causing it to be referred to as "the Western disease". This new number means that autism is much more common as it was thought to be only 5 years ago, affecting over 1,000,000 children in North America.

What is Autism (ASD)?

Autism is a complex development disability that affects a person's ability to communicate and interact with others. The new theory of autism suggests that the brains of people with autism are structurally normal but dysregulated, meaning the symptoms of the disorder might be reversible. This theory suggests that autism is a developmental disorder caused by impaired regulation of a bundle of neutrons in the brain stem that processes sensory signals from all areas of the body.

The Three Main Areas of Difficulty Are:

1. **Impairment in social interaction**

May include:

- Limited use and understanding of non-verbal communication such as facial expressions and gestures.

- Difficulties forming and sustaining friendships.

- Lack of seeking to share enjoyment, interests and activities with other people.

- Difficulties with social and emotional responsiveness.

2. **Impairment in communication**

May include:

- Delayed language development.

- Difficulties in initiating and sustaining conversations.

- Stereotyped and repetitive use of language such as repetitive phrases from television.

- Limited imaginative or make-believe play.

3. **Restrictive and repetitive interests, activities and behaviours**

May include:

- Unusually intense or focused interests.

- Repetitive use of objects, such as repeatedly lining up toys.

- Adherence to non-functional routines such as travelling the same route every day.

- Unusual sensory interests such as sniffing objects, foods or staring at moving objects.

- Sensory sensitivities, including avoidance of everyday sounds.

- Unusual or severely limited interests.

Possible Signs of Autism Spectrum Disorders:

- Trouble with pointing or making meaningful gestures by year 1.

- Cannot speak one word by 16 months.

- Cannot combine two words at 2 years old.

- Does not smile.

- Does not respond to their name.

- Noticeable delays in language or social skills.

- Avoids making eye contact.

- Strongly resists changes in routine.

- Has problems with, or is not interested in playing with toys.

- At times seems to be hearing impaired.

- Has problems interacting with other children or adults.

Secondary Problems:

- Neurological disorders, including epilepsy.

- Gastro-intestinal problems.

- Anxiety and depression.

Children with ASD develop motor, language, cognitive and social skills at different rates from other children at their age.

Autism Spectrum Disorder Is Not:

- Infectious.

- Contagious.

- Caused by vaccines.

- Caused by parental behaviour or parenting style.

Source: National Alliance for Autism Research; Autism Spectrum Australia; Autism Enigma Production Inc.

Facts About Autism:

- Autism now affects 1 in 88 children (1 in 54 boys).

- Autism costs an average family $60,000 per year.

- There is no medical cure for autism.

Source: Autism Speaks

The Mystery of Autism:

- Some 200,000 Canadians are living with autism.

- By the time autism is diagnosed, usually around age 3, the best time for treatment has passed.

- Autism is more common than pediatric cancer, juvenile diabetes and HIV/AIDS combined.

Source: Genome Canada

Authors' Note: Alberta has taken the lead in research into Autism Spectrum Disorder and it is with the kind permission of the Autism Society of Edmonton that we make this chapter available to parents and teachers.

Chapter Two

Autism Spectrum Disorder consists of 5 main types:

1. *Classic autism:* The most severe form, causing significant language delays, social, communication challenges and intellectual disability.

2. *Asperger's syndrome:* Milder form, with some social challenges and unusual behaviours and interests. Can be socially awkward and lack empathy.

3. *Nonspecific pervasive developmental disorder:* Shows some but not all of the symptoms of classic autism.

4. *Rett syndrome:* Marked by poor head growth, it leads to poor verbal skills and repetitive movements.

5. *Childhood disintegrative disorder:* Develops in children who have no symptoms. Can stop talking and socializing.

Source: www.daileymail.co

Of all 5 of these main types of Autism Spectrum Disorder, the type that has the highest rate of bullying incidents is Asperger's syndrome.

Children with Asperger's generally have difficulties in the following areas:

Communication:

- Spoken language—May have difficulty putting thoughts into words, may speak loudly, may correct the language of others, may take what seems to be a long time to react to a question.

- Understanding of language—May have difficulty understanding others (even though he/she speaks well or has or has above average vocabulary), may have difficulty with humor, sarcasm, idioms, abstract language, etc.

- Non-verbal understanding of others—May not remember faces or understand body language, may not be aware of commonly understood social rules.

- Non-verbal self-expression—May not make eye contact, may stare, may make unusual facial expressions or grimaces, may stand too close.

Social Relationships:

- Often have difficulty maintaining relationships with peers the same age.

- May not understand the give and take of social relationships.

- May not understand that others have different thoughts or feelings, or have a different point of view.

Restrictive, Repetitive Interests, Routines, Rituals or Motor Mannerisms (often related to anxiety)

- May flap hands, rock body, etc.

- May insist on doing things in a certain order

- May talk about only one subject.

Additional Common Difficulties:

- Anxiety disorders, including generalized anxiety disorder, phobias, panic attacks or obsessive compulsive disorder.

- Heightened or suppressed emotional states—may become extremely upset, angry, excited or happy; alternatively, may seem unresponsive and withdrawn.

- Sensory irregularities—over-sensitive or under-responsive to sound, light, touch, smell or taste, including difficulties with balance and awareness of his/her body in the space that it occupies.

- Difficulty with change of any kind, transition from one activity to the next, new situations, surprises, disappointments, etc.

- Motor difficulties—may have difficulty learning to print or write.

- Organization—may have difficulty managing personal belongings, homework, planning, etc.

- Learning disabilities—may have a wide range of difficulties including auditory or visual processing, short term memory, etc.

- Attention problems—may have difficulty knowing what he/she is supposed to be focusing on, may have difficulty maintaining focus.

- Depression—some children become depressed at a very young age, many experience depression as they age. Depression may express itself in sadness, crying, sleep difficulties, withdrawing, self-abusive behaviour, or aggression.

Typical Positive Qualities of Children with Asperger's:

- Intelligent and creative

- Committed and loyal in relationships

- Honest

- Logical thinkers

- Advanced knowledge in their areas of interest

- Precise attention to detail

- May have excellent rote memory.

Differences:

Each child diagnosed with Autism Spectrum Disorder is different and each child will be affected differently across each of the many characteristics listed above. An approach which works for one child may not work with another. Children with Autism Spectrum Disorder may:

- Withdraw or be demanding

- Excel academically or have severe learning disabilities

- Withdraw in the face of fear, or become more aggressive

- Display repetitive movements or not display any.

Autism Spectrum Disorder is a complex disorder and behaviour is often misunderstood. What may look like laziness, disrespect or willful deçance, may actually be:

- Anxiety

- Difficulty understanding what has been asked

- Difficulty changing from one activity to the next

- Inability to figure out how to do what has been asked.

Children with ASD may appear to be more competent than they actually are. Over time, they often make significant advances in their development and behaviour. However, the disorder is a lifelong one and it limits the child's functioning and his/her ability to learn and behave in typical ways.

While there is no cure for Autism Spectrum Disorders, we should be helping affected children live full and happy lives, and we should also work with teachers and parents to bring out the best in them.

Characteristics of Autism Spectrum Disorder that Directly Impact the Behaviour of Children:

Children with ASD:

- Have social and emotional development which is normally significantly delayed, for example: a 9-year-old may understand and communicate at a 6-year-old level, or a 15-year-old may be performing at a 10-year-old level, emotionally and socially.

- May not generalize information from one situation to another, even if the situation is only slightly different. For example a "no running" rule may need to be taught for the classroom, re-taught for the hall and re-taught for the library.

- Tend to interpret rules rigidly and may confront those who do not follow the stated rules.

- Tend to have a strong sense of justice, and may confront others on behalf of their friends, or of themselves, for perceived unfairness.

- Often don't know the unwritten rules of different social situations. For example they may speak to a teacher or principal as they would to a classmate, they may speak out of turn, interrupt, tell the teacher he/she is wrong, etc.

- Tend to be very honest. This can be perceived by adults as impertinence or rudeness, though the student has no such intention. Honesty can also get them into difficulties with peers. For example, they may have no understanding of the social consequences of tattling on their peers.

- Often misread nonverbal communication. They may be unaware when someone is furious, bored, tired, sick, etc. Unless the person tells them explicitly.

- May not be able to see another person's point of view and may have no idea how their behaviour affects others. They may not realize when they embarrass their peers, parents, or teachers.

- May have difficulty taking turns, waiting, standing in line, being on the losing team, etc. for reasons related to different characteristics of autism. For example, due to hyper-sensitivity to touch, the student may not be able to tolerate being bumped or jostled by classmates. Due to overwhelming anxiety, the student may not be able to stand still and wait.

- May interpret language literally. For example, when a child is told that he/she will have computer class tomorrow, he/she may become extremely upset when told the next day this will not happen. The child may challenge the teacher, accuse the teacher of lying, or misunderstand the reason for the change.

- May get stuck on a topic and not be able to let it go. For example: a worry, a situation judged by them as unfair, or an anticipated event. They may not be able to move on without assistance.

- "Splintering" of abilities is typical. They may be able to read and understand a book on science, but not a novel. They may be very articulate, but be unable to follow a sequence of instructions.

- They are normally not equipped socially or emotionally to deal with bullying or teasing.

- Depression may become a problem in elementary, junior or senior high school, as academic and social expectations change. They may become ostracized by their peers. They need help gaining peer support and establishing healthy connections.

Some Suggestions for the Classroom:

- Avoid taking the behaviour of autistic children personally. They may have little or no understanding of the impact of their behaviour on others. Their behaviour may be their way of communicating that they are feeling confused, anxious, afraid or overwhelmed.

- Expect unusual or even "outrageous" behaviour and be prepared to respond calmly with clear expectations delivered in short sentences.

- Be prepared to teach basic social rules, such as: you do not touch the teacher's desk without permission.

- Expect inconsistent behaviour and understand that what the child may be able to do one day, he/she may not be capable of doing the next day, or under different conditions.

- **Understand that the child's behaviour is often the result of neurological differences in the way they experience the world. They are not able to change some behaviours, and may need environmental and program accommodations to enable them to experience success in school as well as life.**

- Have available a quiet place for the ASD student to retreat to when his/her experience of the environment becomes overwhelming.

- Seek out other teachers who have worked with ASD to share information and ideas, for support.

- Know as parents we are very supportive of your eëorts and commitment in working with our children and giving them the essential opportunity for an inclusive education.

Bullying Statistics:

According to a survey of parents by the Interactive Autism Network and John Hopkins University researchers:

- 61% of kids with Asperger's have experienced bullying.

- In comparison, 37% of children with autism spectrum disorders have experienced bullying.

- 30% had experienced physical bullying.

- About 50% of parents reported that schoolmates deliberately tried to trigger autistic meltdowns in their children.

- Bullies tend to pick victims they know their classmates won't defend.

- Teasing was the most common form of bullying.

- 73% of their kids experienced taunts.

- Almost half of ASD kids had been deliberately ignored by peers.

- 47% had been called names.

Source: Yahoo News Canada

A child with ASD, because he/she behaves differently, is vulnerable to being excluded, to verbal abuse and to other forms of bullying by peers. The bullying can be extremely subtle, such as making a noise which bothers him/her. Sensitivities to sound can make this situation intolerable.

Children with ASD often want social involvement, but may be socially clumsy, a reality that is not well tolerated by peers, especially as the students grow older. Their developmental delays, emotionally and socially, leave them without essential skills needed to interact with peers.

Suggestions for Intervention

Prevention:

- Alert all school staff to the child's vulnerability to exclusion, verbal abuse, being taken advantage of and other forms of bullying.

- Encourage sympathetic classmates to make eëorts to include the student, or even better, promote the development of a circle of friends.

- Arrange a presentation for the class about Autism Spectrum Disorder and about how the students can be supportive (with the parents' and the student's permission).

- Monitor peer interactions closely, in the classroom as well as outside. A high percentage of bullying occurs in the classroom.

- The child may have difficulty explaining the bullying situation, the sequence of events, etc.

- Provide visual clues, for example: take the child to the gym, have him/her show you what happened, act it out.

Provide Physical Protection:

Put in place a concrete plan of action for when bullying takes place: who the child will talk to and what that person will do to help, and ensure the teachers are part of the plan. Provide the students with direct teaching of the acts of bullying.

Provide Emotional Protection:

- Let the child know that you believe him/her. Children with ASD rarely lie.

- Reassure the child that you will help him/her and that it is ok to ask for help.

- Children with ASD may need intensive help with bullying all throughout school.

Children with ASD are often naïve and unsophisticated. They may need protection well into adulthood, from those who may want to take advantage of them.

Many children with ASD have anxiety disorders and/or depression. Unresolved bullying can lead to emotional and/or psychological breakdown.

Source: Autism Society of Edmonton

Part Three

Issues that Concern Today's Youth

Chapter One

Suicide

How you can help:

- Listen and hear. Of vital importance to a person in an emotional crisis is having someone available who will listen carefully to what he or she is saying. Avoid false reassurances that "everything will be okay" and never demean suicidal expressions. Don't be judgmental or moralizing.

- Be supportive. Communicate your concern.

- Be sensitive to the relative seriousness of thoughts and feelings. Inquire directly about thoughts of suicide. If we don't respond to the seriousness of the situation, they may interpret our reactions as not caring. Suicide is a topic that makes us all uncomfortable, but we must face it with open, honest communication. When a person speaks of clear-cut self-destructive plans, they are usually contemplating this course of action. Take any mention of suicide seriously, even if expressed in a calm voice.

- Trust your own judgment. If you do believe someone is in danger of committing suicide, act on your beliefs. Don't let others mislead you into ignoring warning signals. **Be an alarmist.**

- Tell others. Share your knowledge with the counselor and/or school psychologist. Don't worry about breaking a vow of secrecy. You may have to reveal a secret to save a life.

- Stay with a suicidal person. Don't leave them alone if you think there is immediate danger. Call upon whoever can be of assistance.

- Be concerned about previous attempts. A student who has tried to take their own life is a high risk to try again. If you are aware that someone has done so, tell the counselor and/or psychologist. Make sure they know.

What to Look For:

Verbal Signs: "I wish I were dead." "No one cares whether I live or die." "Things would be better if I weren't here."

Behaviour Clues: Alcohol or drug abuse, previous attempts, giving away possessions, making a will, sudden change in behaviour (e.g. a quiet student becomes talkative, friendly student becomes quiet), significant drop in grades, risk-taking behaviour resulting in accident or injuries.

Situational Clues: End of a serious relationship, divorce or death of a parent, family financial difficulties, moving to a new location (or other significant stresses among family members).

Syndromic Clues: Social isolation, depression, disorientation and changes in sleeping and/or eating patterns, dissatisfaction (e.g. constant complaining and helpless/hopeless feelings).

Common stressors experienced by adolescents who attempt suicide:

- Breakup with a boyfriend or girlfriend

- Trouble with a sibling

- Dramatic change in parents' finances

- Loss of a close friend

- Change of school

- Injury or illness

- Trouble with a teacher and/or failing grades

- Increased arguments with friends

Questions concerning suicide:

1. Does almost everyone at least think of suicide during his/her lifetime?

2. Is there a certain time of the year when more suicides occur, for example, during holidays?

3. Do losses of loved ones or relationships have much to do with youth suicide?

4. Will teenagers talk about their suicidal thoughts?

5. What methods do boys use most often?

6. Can students who talk about suicide be classified as low-risk?

7. Has the rate of youth suicide really increased that much, or is it just being publicized more widely?

8. Is there a certain type of student who is at risk for suicide?

9. How should someone respond to a suicidal student?

10. Why do drugs and alcohol play such a large role in youth suicide?

11. Can the suicide of one adolescent "trigger" the suicide of another?

12. Is a student who runs away from home at a risk for committing suicide?

13. Will adolescents who are prevented from killing themselves once keep trying until they succeed?

Answers:

1. **Yes.** Many of us gives it some thought.

2. **No.** There is a slight increase in the spring, but there is no one time of the year, such as Christmas, when a disproportionate number of suicides occur.

3. **Yes.** Students who have experienced numerous losses may feel helpless and hopeless and turn to suicide. We also must take the breakup of adolescent romance seriously, because such breakups often precipitate suicide attempts.

4. **Yes.** If someone they trust provides them with an opportunity to do so. The key is to let them talk and reflect their feelings. Their suicidal thoughts should not be dismissed or minimized.

5. Guns account for approximately 60% of boys' suicides. Gun safety programs and convincing families not to have guns accessible in the home are keys to prevention.

6. **No.** Students who talk about it are at risk. If they do not receive prompt attention, they may act out their suicidal thoughts.

7. The rate has increased 300% since the 1950's.

8. **No.** There is no type. Depression has long been associated with youth suicide. Recently, emphasis has also been placed on conduct disorders and substance abuse as associated problems.

9. Respond openly, honestly and directly. Let the student know that you care. Give him or her permission to talk about suicidal thoughts.

10. Drugs and alcohol impair contact with reality and contribute to a teenager's acting on suicidal thoughts. Alcohol and drugs are also depressants and make young people further depressed.

11. **Yes.** Adolescents are more likely to imitate the suicide of another than adults. Factors believed to be involved are impulsiveness, impressionability and striving for recognition or glamorization through suicidal actions.

12. **Yes.** Research has shown that from 20% to 25% of adolescents who run away from home attempt suicide.

13. **No.** Most attempts are situational in nature. The adolescent who is stopped and who gets professional help is unlikely to try again.

Levels of Suicide Intervention and Specific Activities:

Primary Intervention

- Annual in-service training session for all school faculty. Emphasize the warning signs and referral procedures with handouts.

- Annual training provided to counselors and nurses.

- Training provided to teachers in subjects such as health, psychology and sociology.

- Presentations to student groups.

- Community and school-based presentations for parents, emphasizing mental health and suicide prevention.

- Articles written on suicides and/or prevention, published in local newspapers, sent to the Parent Support Group.

- Group counseling provided weekly to "at risk" students.

- Establishment of teen help-line programs.

Secondary Intervention

- Assessment of the severity level of the students' suicidal thoughts or actions.

- Notification to the parent of a suicidal student.

- Activities to assist faculty and students through the grieving process immediately following a suicide, and to minimize the contagious effects of the suicide.

- Support media attention that downplays the suicide method employed and instead publicizes where to get help.

- Contact with the parents of the student who committed suicide to offer sympathy, assistance with surviving siblings, and coordination of services between the school and family.

Tertiary Intervention

- Long-term follow-up of those who have been affected by the suicide of a friend or relative.

- Awareness of anniversary dates of losses and the birthdays of significant others who have committed suicide, and provision of support for those who need it at those difficult times.

Major Symptoms of Depression

- Withdrawal from friends and social activities.

- Loss of joy in life and a bleak outlook for the future.

- Changes in sleeping and eating habits.

- Preoccupation with death.

- Increased somatic complaints.

- Concentration problems with regard to schoolwork.

- Frequent mood changes.

- Uncharacteristic emotional or rebellious outbursts.

- Low self-esteem and lack of confidence in abilities and decision-making capabilities.

- Significant weight loss or gain.

- Decreased attention to physical appearance.

Chapter Two

Drugs

What are drugs?

Drugs are substances taken to change the way that the mind or body works. There are four categories:

1. Stimulants

2. Depressants

3. Hallucinogens

4. Cannabis

Seven major reasons why people take drugs:

1. Out of curiosity.

2. Because they feel emotional pressures such as loneliness or depression.

3. They feel pressured to do so by the people around them.

4. They want to ęt in with friends.

5. Because drugs are easy to get.

6. They have used them before.

7. They do not feel right without them. They are drug dependent.

Facts:

- Over 60% of all people killed in drunk-driving accidents are teenagers. Traffic accidents are the leading cause of teenage deaths. Over half of all traffic accidents resulting in death involve alcohol.

- Over half of all children in grade 7 have tried alcohol or some other drug and over 90% by grade 12.

- Alcoholism, between the ages of 9 and 12, once unheard of, is becoming increasingly common.

- Addiction is hereditary. Studies show that sons of alcoholic fathers have a 4 to 5 times greater chance of becoming alcoholics themselves.

- Alcohol and tobacco are the two drugs used most by young people. Boys are generally bigger drug users than girls, with the exception of tobacco. Girls are much more dependent on cigarettes.

- After alcohol and tobacco, marijuana is the most widely used drug by both young people and adults.

Marijuana . . .
what it is and how it affects you . . .

- Your perceptions of time and space change. Time may seem to pass slowly and distances become distorted.

- Your balance may become impaired.

- You might feel outgoing and talkative, and laugh more.

- You might not be able to remember things that just happened. It may be harder to think clearly and perform certain tasks, like homework.

- If you're pregnant, the more cannabis you smoke, the more likely your baby will have problems, such as low birth weight.

- Cannabis is more powerful today than it was 20 years ago because growers have developed plants that contain more THC than before.

- Marijuana, hash and hash oil all come from the same plant called "cannabis sativa". All three contains THC, a chemical that changes the way you think, feel and act.

- THC is short for "delta-9-tetrahydrocannabinol". It is responsible for the "high" that changes a person's mood and perception.

- Cannabis can be smoked or eaten but it can't be taken with a needle, because it doesn't dissolve in water.

- A common slang name for a marijuana cigarette is a joint. Street names: pot, hash, weed, dope, honey oil (hash oil), ganja.

- When cannabis is smoked, the THC reaches the brain faster than when it is eaten.

- People who use cannabis every day and quit suddenly may have problems sleeping or become anxious, irritable or nervous without the drug. They may also have an upset stomach. These symptoms, if they occur, rarely last more than a few days.

What Problems Does Drug Abuse Cause?

Drug abuse causes health problems and can lead to sickness and physical damage to our body. Smoking marijuana or tobacco has a high likelihood of causing cancer. Abusing alcohol can cause damage to the liver. Sniffing drugs can ruin the inside of your nose.

Drugs taken with needles can cause infections, serum hepatitis or collapsing veins. Even more frightening is the possibility of contracting AIDS associated with needles. **These are only a few of the health risks that are related to the use of drugs.**

Drug abuse can cause personal, social and mental problems. It can lead to problems of addiction and loss of motivation. Many will turn to drugs to avoid normal feelings of being depressed.

Once you are in the habit of using drugs, it is hard to stop the habit. When a drug user's body gets so used to a drug that it cannot function without it, it's "physically dependent" on the drug. Without the drug, the user will go through "withdrawal". Withdrawal can be uncomfortable or it can be very painful.

A person can be emotionally addicted to drugs before a physical addiction occurs. Emotional addiction makes it very difficult for the person to view his/her drug use objectively. Even though their drug use is replacing things that used to be important in their lives, they do not recognize it as abuse since there are no physical symptoms.

The transition of values might seem like a natural change in their life.

Tips on Being Drug-Free

- Make a personal commitment to live drug-free. This can be a silent pledge to yourself or a formal pledge between you and a group of your peers.

- Establish friendships with others who want to live drug-free. Join a youth prevention group. Seek support for your choice and help others do the same.

- Saying "NO" to drugs means saying "YES" to drug-free alternatives.

- Find a good role model who doesn't use drugs. It can be a family member, a popular celebrity or someone such as your favourite teacher or sports coach. The right role models must believe in a no-use rule about alcohol and other drugs for minors, and also model appropriate behaviour themselves.

- Develop a strong relationship with your parents. Let them know what concerns you have. Talk about the drug issue. They want to be part of your lives, so why not let them in.

- Learn up-to-date and accurate adverse health effects of alcohol and drugs (non-medicinal purposes) on the body. Being well-informed will make it easier to say "NO" to drugs.

- Practice techniques of resisting peer pressure. Role-play with a younger brother or sister, a friend, or an adult. This will help you to react negatively without hesitation in a real-life situation.

- Look at the long-term consequences of your actions. Ask yourself these two questions which will help you say "NO": "Would me saying "YES" to my friends request breaking the law?" and "Would I do this in front of my parents, teachers or other responsible adults in my life?"

- Be an individual. This means not going along with the crowd when they do something you don't agree with. Be a thermostat, not a thermometer: grab control of your environment before it controls you.

Be proud of your drug-free choice and realize that you are great just the way you are.

Chapter Three

Alcohol

Uses of Alcohol

Alcohol is one of the more readily available drugs. It is a depressant, a drug that slows down the central nervous system. The active ingredient in alcohol is a chemical called ethyl alcohol, which, taken in large doses, is poison to the body. When a person drinks, the liver filters alcohol from the blood stream and eliminates it from the body. The liver can filter about one ounce of alcohol per hour. If someone drinks at a faster rate, the person becomes intoxicated or drunk.

People are consuming alcohol at a younger age each year. Today, the average age of those starting to use alcohol is 12.5. Research shows that the younger a person is when he or she starts to drink alcohol, the greater are the chances that the person will develop into a chronic alcoholic. Alcoholism in adolescence develops very rapidly, with some teenagers becoming alcoholics within six months of taking their first drink.

Negative Effects of Alcohol Use:

- Damage to brain and liver cells (cirrhosis).

- Impaired thinking. You say things you don't mean or wish you hadn't said.

- Arrest, if bought or used under-age or while driving.

- Dependence on alcohol to relax.

- Alcoholism.

- Slurred speech, slowed reflexes.

- Expensive to purchase.

- Nausea, vomiting.

- Loss of non-drinking friends.

- Inflammation of the stomach.

- Weakening of heart muscle.

- Cancers of the esophagus, mouth, pharynx, larynx, liver; possible cause of breast and colorectal cancer.

- Loss of brain cells.

How Alcohol Affects You

- Too much alcohol can cause a hangover: headache, nausea, shakiness and even vomiting afterwards.

- Alcohol use increases the risk of high blood pressure and related illness for both men and women. It may increase the risk of breast cancer in women.

- People who have been drinking heavily often have withdrawal symptoms when they stop drinking, or cut down. The symptoms may include nervousness, sleep problems, tremors (the "shakes"), seizures and hallucinations.

Alcohol Fact Sheet

Myth: Alcohol is not really a drug.

Fact: Alcohol is a serious and potentially dangerous drug. Many people die every year from alcohol poisoning (overdose), as well as from consequences of long-term, heavy drinking.

Myth: Beer and wine are not as bad as "hard" alcohol.

Fact: The effects of alcohol do not depend on whether you are drinking beer, wine or liquor, but on how much a person drinks, the situation in which drinking takes place, over what period of time, and other factors. One bottle of beer or one glass of wine has roughly the same amount as one mixed drink.

Myth: The people with real alcohol problems live on skid row.

Fact: Most people with alcohol problems are ordinary people from every walk of life. They hold jobs, go to school, have families. People who drink even relatively low amounts of alcohol can experience problems that affect their families, friends, co-workers and others. Impaired driving accidents or work related injuries are just a few examples.

Drinking Influences

- Social Pressure: Pressure from family members, friends, role models or other peers who drink alcohol.

- Advertising Pressure: Advertising links drinking alcohol with attractive people, lifestyles and attitudes.

- Rebel: You want to defy authority and take a risk.

- Experimenting: You want to see what it is like.

- Dealing with Stress: Some people get used to drinking when they get stressed out, but drinking puts extra stress on your body.

Drinking and Driving

The term "Blood Alcohol Concentration" or BAC refers to the amount of alcohol in a person's body. BAC can be determined by measuring the weight of alcohol in a fixed volume of blood. BAC can also be measured in a person's breath by using an instrument called a "breathalyzer". Breath tests are just as accurate as blood tests for measuring BAC.

BAC is important because it relates to how much you drink, how strongly alcohol affects you, how much greater the risk of being involved in an accident, and how close you may be to breaking the law.

RIDE programs are used extensively when drunk drivers are more likely to be driving a vehicle. The deaths and accidents caused by these drivers place a heavy burden on all of us: unnecessary loss of life, severe injuries, large increases in auto insurance.

Designated drivers save lives.

Chapter Four

Tobacco

The Facts:

- Tobacco is the legal consumer product that kills when used exactly as intended.

- There is no safe level of tobacco consumption.

- About 3,000 people in Ontario die annually from inhaling other people's smoke.

- Tobacco advertising is banned in Canada.

- A pack per day cost a cigarette smoker approximately $3,000 per year.

- It takes a teenager less than 5 cigarettes to be addicted to nicotine.

- The equivalent of one tree is burned for every 300 cigarettes manufactured.

Children and Tobacco:

- Most smokers in Canada start as children who are initiated into tobacco addiction, on average, at age 12.

- 13 is the average age at which teens start smoking on a daily basis.

- 75% of young smokers become addicted users before age 17.

- Children under age 19 purchase cigarettes worth more than an estimated $400 million and consume 2 billion or more cigarettes each year.

- According to Canadian surveys that test retailer compliance with tobacco restraint laws, many stores will sell cigarettes to minors.

- 18,000 to 20,000 out of every 100,000 smokers now age 15 will die from tobacco related diseases before they reach age 70—about 8 times the total number of deaths projected for this group from other drug abuse, car accidents, suicide, murder and AIDS combined.

Statistics Tell the Story:

- Incidence of regular smoking in the 15-to 19-year-old age group has declined but the numbers still remain alarmingly high despite the advances in tobacco use prevention. One out of 8 Canadian children smokes. Girls are now more likely to smoke than boys.

- In households where both parents smoke, 33% of teens aged 15-19 also are smokers. In households with one adult smoker, this percentage drops to 21%, and with no adult smokers it decreases to 13%.

Pre-Indicators of a Young Smoker:

- Low self-esteem;

- Poor academic record;

- Less physically active;

- Working part or fulltime;

- Peer group smokes;

- Parents or siblings are smokers;

- Low-income family;

- Less-educated family.

Tobacco Advertising

The World Health Organization estimates that tobacco will prematurely kill 200 million people who are now children, and eventually wipe out 500 million in the world.

Tobacco advertisements are banned in Canada but tobacco companies continue to spend a lot of money to promote their products. For example, one tobacco company sponsors a number of jazz festivals throughout the country that bear the cigarette brand's

72 name. The tobacco industry relies upon the promotion of special events to attract new teen "addicts" in order to survive.

Current tobacco ads target Women, Minorities, Children and other select groups. Tobacco companies do this by associating cigarettes with popular themes such as risk—taking, glamour, sex, and financial and personal success. The models in cigarettes ads are portrayed as cool, beautiful and smart. Actors are paid to smoke on-screen while making movies.

What cigarette manufacturers don't want you to know: Janet Sachman, Lucky Strikes' former cover girl, has had her larynx removed due to throat cancer. Wayne McLaren, the former Marlboro Man, has died of lung cancer. David Goerlite, former Winston model, has suffered a stroke.

Smoking is still increasing around the world. It is likely to grow by about 2% per year through at least the next decade. The bottom line is: Children are now the primary target because the tobacco industry thinks they can take advantage of them. Do you think this shameful exploitation should be allowed to continue? Be Aware!

Smoking is a negative peer pressure situation. The main reason young people begin smoking is because their peers do, and that's not a good reason to do many things. The negative effects of smoking can be permanent. The real way to act grown-up is to act responsibly, and smoking is not acting responsibly. Remember that you can always just say "NO!"

Preventing Tobacco Problems

Tobacco is an extreme health hazard that is a "gateway drug". It serves as an entry point to a lifestyle that eventually or perhaps concurrently, includes the use of alcohol and other drugs that have the potential for abuse. All tobacco use is harmful, even if you do not die from it. Tobacco smoke is also harmful to developing fetuses and to nonsmokers. One of three who continue to smoke in adulthood will die prematurely from smoking related illnesses.

It is important to start tobacco prevention early, because the tobacco industry starts early in aiming its $6,000,000,000 a year advertising and promotional programs at children, as they attempt to replace smokers who die or quit with young ones who are easily misled.

Why Do People Smoke?

People start smoking because they see it as meeting certain needs. People also start because they are curious about the effects of tobacco. They believe it will alter their mood. And because smoking is forbidden, they want to rebel against or defy their parents.

The Addiction Process

The dangers of this drug are underestimated. Children should be told that nobody starts chewing or smoking tobacco, or using any other drug, expecting to get addicted. Everyone believes that they can get the beneęts without the harm. This belief is wrong—dead wrong. Regular use soon results in addiction.

Five stages of tobacco use:

1. Forming attitudes, beliefs and expectations about what you get from smoking.

2. Trying smoking, the first two or three times that cigarettes are used.

3. Experimentation, which involves repeated but irregular use.

4. Regular use, which means at least twice a week.

5. Dependence.

Changes Your Body Goes Through When You Quit

Within 20 minutes of your last cigarette:

- Blood pressure may drop to normal level;

- Pulse rate drops to normal level;

- Skin temperature of hands and feet increases to normal.

8 hours:

- Carbon monoxide level in blood drops;

- Oxygen level in blood increases.

24 hours:

- May reduce chance of heart attack.

48 hours:

- Nerve endings may regroup;

- Ability to smell and taste enhanced.

72 hours:

- Bronchial tubes relax, if undamaged this will make breathing easier;

- Lung capacity increases.

2 weeks to 3 months:

- Circulation improves;

- Walking becomes easier;

- Lung function may increase up to 20%.

1 month to 9 months:

- Coughing, sinus congestion, fatigue, shortness of breath may decrease markedly over a number of weeks;

- Potential for cilia to regroup in lungs, increasing ability to handle mucus, clean the lungs, reduce infection;

- Body's overall energy level increases.

5 years:

- Lung cancer death rate for average smoker (one pack a day) decreases from 137 per 100,000 to 72 per 100,000.

10 years:

- Precancerous cells are replaced;

- Other cancers such as those of the mouth, larynx, esophagus, bladder, kidney and pancreas decrease (there are approximately 50 chemicals in tobacco smoke that cause cancer).

Chapter Five

Peer Pressure

Students are faced with inevitable peer pressure, so it is not a question of just saying "NO"; it is a matter of how to refuse situations with which they feel uncomfortable. You often hear about children and peer pressure, but we should recognize that conformity is a problem for all age groups in this culture. Even many adults drink, use drugs, and engage in many other activities just to be accepted by their peers.

One person may often be right when somebody else is wrong, and it takes unusual courage to stick to your guns when you're in a definite minority. Will you give in when everyone else says you're wrong? In other words, will you give in, in order to be liked and included, or will you do what you know is right? When do you give in? When do you make a stand?

One task of school-aged children is to learn that it is okay to believe and act differently from one's friends. Children are learning this skill when they resist peer pressure. The pressure may be something illegal, like drugs or stealing; something dishonest, like lying or cheating; or due to different values, like partying or status-symbol clothes. In dealing with peer pressure, a direct approach usually works best. Four approaches are: be blunt, refer to a parent, get an ally, and bargain.

Be Blunt

One way to combat pressure to do something illegal is to call it by its legal term. For example, if a friend wants you to take a candy bar without paying for it, reply, "You're crazy. That's shoplifting, I could get arrested. I can do without that kind of trouble." And then leave.

Refer to a Parent

Another way to resist illegal acts is to say, "I can't do that. My dad (mom) would ground me." If the friends say that they would not find out, insist, "You don't know my dad, he finds out everything. He would be very angry." And again leave. Most parents would quickly agree to support any excuse or reason kids give when they won't do something illegal or questionable.

Get an Ally

Peers often try to make others feel as though everyone else does "it", whether "it" is smoking, cheating on a test, or something else you know is wrong. With this approach, you name someone else who won't do "it". For example, "I'm not going to. It's not right. Terry and I are going to do . . . . instead."

Bargain

If you have something (an item or skill) someone needs or wants, you could use this to strike a bargain. This way, you are preventing them from doing something you know is wrong and you are showing them the strength of your convictions.

Peer Influences

Everyone wants to have friends that you share common things with. A peer group is a group who shares common things. Having friends is necessary and an important part of learning to become an adult.

As you get older, you begin to spend more time with people your own age. Then you start to keep company with different groups of friends (peer groups) in and out of school. "Fitting in" with a group is very important. Your peer group gives you feelings of belonging and identity, and it oěers you support. Your peer group also affects your decision-making and puts pressure on you to be the same as the others in the group.

Most of the time you probably don't even realize that your friends have such an effect on your thoughts and actions. Group pressures can be helpful, but sometimes they are not. When it comes to smoking, drinking and using drugs, some of you will try them because your friends are trying them. It is not easy to say "NO" when you want to fit in.

These will be hard situations for you to deal with. Just remember that you can think and act for yourself. You can make your own decisions and avoid problems. You can help your friends and they can help you. **Together, you can make the right choices.**

Chapter Six

Abuse

Sexual Abuse

Physical characteristics may suggest that a child has been or currently is a victim of sexual abuse. Lack of physical evidence of the abuse only means that the act did not leave any. A child, depending on their age, may be the victim of an ongoing series of sexual acts without exhibiting any physical signs.

Possible signs include:

- Difficulty in walking or sitting;

- Torn, stained, or bloody underwear;

- Genital/anal bruises or bleeding;

- Frequent urinary tract or yeast infections;

- Pain when urinating;

- Pregnancy;

- Loss of appetite;

- Chronic and unexplained sore throats.

Behaviour Indications of Sexual Abuse

Fear:

Fear is the most common initial reaction. For that reason, the child who expresses fear (and/or anxiety) for no apparent reason should be given special attention until the cause of the problem is determined.

Inability to Trust:

Because of the betrayal that the child has suffered at the hands of an adult, and because the child has been made to feel helpless by the adult, the child becomes severely limited in his/her ability to trust. This may impair their future relationships in many ways.

Anger and Hostility:

Children are rarely able to express their anger towards an assailant, and as a result it is often displaced onto others. However, in a few cases (usually those that involve extra-familial abuse) the child does find an opportunity to release their anger toward the abuser.

Inappropriate Sexual Behaviour:

Sexually abused children may attempt to show or tell others what happened by doing or acting out what was done to them. A child may also attempt to gain a sense of mastery over the trauma by repetition of the events. For example: child victims of sexual assault (especially male victims) may attempt to undo their feelings of helplessness by doing to other children what was done to them—a manifestation of "identification with the aggressor".

Depression:

Because of not being able to express their feelings of helpless rage for what was done to them, abused children may become clinically depressed, showing signs of emotional constriction and flat or bland reactions.

Guilt or Shame:

Since young children are by nature egocentric, they may mistakenly accept responsibility for other people's actions towards them. This tendency, when added to the molester's attempts to shift blame onto the victim, often results in the child's experiencing intense feelings of guilt and/or shame for what has happened to them.

Problems in School:

A sudden drop in school performance may be a symptom of sexual abuse. In some cases though, performance does not falter because the child may find security in the structure of the school environment.

Somatic Complaints:

Many sexually abused children internalize their trauma and may demonstrate varied somatic disorders such as headaches or stomachaches that have no organic cause.

Sleep Disturbances:

Frequently, sexually abused children experience difficulty in sleeping, fear of sleeping alone, nightmares, or even terror.

Eating Disorders:

Some victims of sexual abuse exhibit eating disorders, as evidenced by a sudden marked increase or decrease in appetite or the hoarding of food. A clinician should be especially observant when treating anorexia or bulimia in adolescents because those symptoms may mask trauma caused by sexual assault.

Phobic or Avoidant Behaviour:

Child victims may display a wide range of avoidant behaviour from agoraphobia to school phobia to the fear of someone who even slightly resembles the molester in appearance.

Regressive Behaviour:

Children may become regressive as a result of sexual trauma. Hence, cases of regression that are not readily explained should be checked carefully for possible evidence of such abuse.

Self-Destructive Behaviour or Accident-Proneness:

These may become outlets for the child's feelings of guilt or shame. Many child molesters' victims feel damaged or worthless, and their actions take this form of self-abuse.

Running Away:

Older children may attempt to cope with sexual abuse by running away from home, which only compounds their dilemma.

When is it Rape?

1. A couple attending college break up. They have been intimate for years, engaging in various forms of sex. One week after they separate, the male arrives at the female's apartment intoxicated and states that they are going to have sex. The female insists that the relationship is over; however, the male gets angry, punches the wall and demands sex. The female knows that he will not hit her and therefore is not frightened for her own safety but gives in, and they engage in sexual relations.

2. On a third date, the male puts double shots of alcohol in his date's drink. She is not an experienced drinker and passes out while they are engaged in heavy petting. The male proceeds to have intercourse with her.

3. A couple has been dating for a few weeks. They both have had several drinks and are intoxicated. They engage in heavy petting and the girl responds physically but says, "please darling, no". The male continues his sexual advances and the girl continues to respond physically but also continues to say "no". They finally engage in intercourse.

Is any of the above acquaintance rape? Why? Who is responsible in these situations? Are both parties at fault?

The above scenarios should be discussed by parents and their adolescent children. Rape is a serious crime and the results could very well ruin lives.

Consequences of Rape:

Fear and Anxiety:

These are the most common reactions to the crime of rape. Burnam conducted a survey of 3,132 households and found that rape victims reported significantly higher levels of phobias and panic disorders than non-victims did. Rape victims suffer a higher level of anxiety than victims of other crimes.

Post-Traumatic Stress Disorder:

Post-traumatic stress disorder is deęned as the development of characteristic symptoms following a psychologically distressing event that is outside the range of usual human experience. The characteristic symptoms involve re-experiencing the traumatic event, avoidance of stimuli associated with the event or numbing of general responsiveness, and increased agitation.

Rape Crisis Syndrome:

This is similar to PTSD. Rape crisis syndrome occurs when the victim experiences feelings of shame, humiliation, disjointedness, anger, inability to concentrate and withdrawal.

Depression:

A number of studies have found that rape victims suffer from depression as a result of their experiences, with classifications ranging from moderate to severely depressed.

Loss of Self-esteem:

The issue of self-blame on the part of the rape victim has been commented on by a number of authorities. However, no conclusive study indicates that rape victims, as a class, suffer lower self-esteem than victims of other crimes.

Research shows, however, that there were long-term problems with self-esteem in rape victims. It is also clear that this is an area that needs further study.

Social Adjustment:

Victims of rape often suffer from economic, social and leisure adjustment. Studies indicate that marital and family adjustments may be more difficult for rape victims as they try to move forward with their lives.

Sexual Functioning:

Although it is clear that rape is now accepted as physical assault in which sex is used to dominate or control the victim, women who have been raped report continuing problems. Sexual dysfunction is one of the most long-lasting effects of rape, with the most common reaction by these victims being the avoidance of sex.

Other Psychological Reactions to Rape:

Other psychological problems may arise as a result of rape. These include, but are not limited to, obsessive compulsive disorders, anger, hostility, fatigue and confusion.

Although the physical act of rape may last minutes, hours, or, in some cases, days, the effects and consequences to the victims may linger for months, years or a lifetime. Being raped is only the beginning of the suffering that the victim will endure.

Some Unsettling Facts about Rape:

- Ninety-eight percent of rape victims will never see their attackers apprehended, convicted or incarcerated.

- Fifty-four percent of all rape charges result in either a dismissal or an acquittal.

- A rape prosecution is more than twice as likely as a murder prosecution to be dismissed, and thirty percent more likely to be dismissed than a robbery.

- Approximately one in ten rapes reported to the police results in time served in prison; one in one hundred convicted rapists is sentenced to more than one year in prison.

- Almost one quarter of convicted rapists are not sentenced to prison but are, instead, released on probation.

These frightening statistics show that more needs to be done to support the victims of such a crime.

Date Rape Drugs
How does it happen?

Victims have had drugs unsuspectingly slipped into their drinks at bars, clubs, and social events for the purpose of reducing their resistance to sexual advances. Once the individual is incapacitated, they are sexually assaulted. Placed in a helpless or unconscious state, they can't escape, resist or call for help.

What is Rohypnol?

Rohypnol is the brand name of Flunitrazepam (a Benz diazepam). It is a sedative which is ten times stronger than valium. Similar in size and shape to aspirin, the pill is a small white tablet that is single or cross-scored on one side and has the word "Roche" and a circled number 1 or 2 on the other side.

Rohypnol dissolves easily in juice, coëee, carbonated and alcoholic beverages. It is colourless, odourless and tasteless when dissolved in any liquid.

The effects of this drug are enhanced when mixed with alcohol, causing sedation, loss of inhibitions, relaxation, blackouts and amnesia. It can also cause respiratory depression, comas **and even death**.

The drug takes effect in about 20 minutes and the effects may last for up to 8-10 hours.

Signs and Symptoms: Quick Intoxication / Drowsiness / Disorientation / Impaired Judgement and Co-ordination / Memory Loss / Hot and Cold Flashes / Nausea / Difficulty in Speaking and Moving.

Street Names: Roffes / Ropies / Ruffies / R2 / Rib / Roaches / Roachies / Mind erasers / Stupeę / Trip-and-fall, and others.

Other Date Rape Drugs:

GHB, which is short for gamma hydroxybutyric, is also known as Bedtime Scoop, Cherry Meth, Easy Lay, Energy Drink, G, Gamma 10, Liquid Ecstasy, Liquid X, Vita-G, and others.

Ketamine, also known as Black Hole, Bump, Cat Valium, green, Jet, K, Kit Kat, Special K, Super Acid, and others.

Source: www.medicinenet.com

Scopolamine (Burundanga) imported from Colombia, it blocks memory and causes submissive behaviour.

Source: *The Devil to Pay*, Harold Robbins and Junius Podrug, A Forge Book, 2006, p. 256.

If Date Rape Happens To You!

- Tell someone you trust.

- Get medical attention A.S.A.P

- Try to collect a urine sample in a clear container in the first 24 hours if you are sexually assaulted. (This may be your only evidence linking the drug to the crime.)

- Don't destroy any of the evidence by showering or washing. Do not disturb anything in the area where the assault occurred.

- Report the incident to the police, your local rape crisis centre, or the hospital emergency department.

- Talk to a counselor for support. Your emotional and physical health is important.

- Believe in yourself. No one invites, causes or deserves to be sexually assaulted.

- What happened to you is a criminal offence, you are not to blame.

How to Avoid Becoming a Victim:

- Do not accept open drinks at parties, particularly from strangers. If you are drinking from a bottle, open it yourself or watch the bartender do it.

- Never leave your drink unattended. If you ask someone to watch it, make sure it is someone you trust.

- Be aware of what is happening around you. Be suspicious of persons who try to handle your drink or insist that you take a drink provided by them.

- Never leave a bar or club with someone you have just met, especially if you are feeling intoxicated.

- If you believe you have ingested a drug, seek medical attention immediately.

- Don't drink anything that has an unusual taste or appearance, i.e. salty taste, has excessive foam or residue.

- Do not mix drugs and alcohol.

Physical Abuse

Indicators:

- Unexplained bruises or welts that may be in various stages of healing, or in clusters of unusual patterns, or on several different areas.

- Unexplained burns in shape of a cigarette, rope, iron, or caused by immersion which may appear sock—or glove-like.

- Unexplained lacerations to mouth, lips, arms, legs or torso.

- Unexplained skeletal injuries, stiff swollen joints or multiple or spiral fractures.

- Missing or loosened teeth.

- Human bite marks.

- Bald spots.

- Unexplained abrasions.

- Appearance of injuries after school absence, weekends or vacations.

Behaviour Indicators:

- Easily frightened or fearful of adults and/or parents, physical contact, or when other children cry.

- Destructive to self and/or others.

- Extremes of behaviour: aggressive or withdrawn.

- Poor social relations.

- Learning problems, poor academic performance, short attention span, delayed language development.

- Runaway or delinquent behaviour.

- Reporting unbelievable reasons for injuries.

- Complains of soreness or moves awkwardly, accident-prone.

- Wears clothing that is clearly meant to cover the body when not appropriate for weather conditions or activities.

- Seems to be afraid to go home.

<u>Signs that a Woman may be in an Abusive Relationship:</u>

- She is not active in social activities or inexplicably withdraws from them after having been an active participant.

- She has no close friends of her own. She seldom invites people to her home, or when she does, visitors get subtle clues that they must leave before her spouse returns.

- She appears nervous and will never accept an invitation without checking first with her spouse.

- She seldom has any cash and has "forgotten" her checkbook, but may have a credit card with her.

- She wears heavy makeup or sunglasses, even indoors. Her wardrobe includes scarves, turtleneck sweaters, long sleeves and slacks.

- She has "accidents" at home.

- At her place of employment she receives and places many phone calls from/to her spouse.

- She and her spouse have frequent changes of residence that seem unrelated to employment requirements.

<u>Child Neglect</u>

<u>Indications:</u>

No single set of factors establishes a clearly deemed line dividing neglect and poor parenting. Any list must be viewed with caution. However, any professional who observes certain characteristics in young children should be suspicious. At the very least, professionals need to reassure themselves of the welfare of the child. On the other hand, further checking may indicate a situational fact pattern that can or will cure itself without the intervention of public agencies.

Certain physical acts by children should alert teachers, nurses, social workers, and others to look for the reasons for these actions. Individual symptoms may appear and, in many instances, may be simply the result of normal childhood activities. However, if more than one of these symptoms persist, the professional should begin to look for a possible pattern of neglect.

Physical Indicators of Neglect

- Poor growth pattern;

- Constant hunger, malnutrition;

- Poor hygiene, strong body odour, and lice;

- Inappropriate clothing;

- Constant fatigue, falling asleep in class;

- Consistent lack of supervision, especially for long periods of time or in potentially dangerous conditions;

- Unexplained bruises or injuries;

- Unattended physical problems or medical needs such as lack of proper immunizations, gross dental problems, the need for glasses/hearing aids.

Professionals should be alert to physical indications of neglect and look for indications that may signal a child has been neglected by their parents.

Characteristics of Parents Who Neglect Their Children

- Inability to plan: They lack the ability to establish goals, objectives and direction. May also have low frustration levels and little ability to delay gratification.

- Lack of Knowledge: They have little or no knowledge of their children's needs, limited housekeeping and cooking skills, etc.

- Lack of Judgment: May leave a young child alone and unsupervised.

- Lack of Motivation: These parents lack energy, have little desire to learn, and no other standard of comparison. They are apathetic in that they are withdrawn an feel that nothing is worth doing.

Characteristics of Children Who Have Been Emotionally Neglected

- Clingy and indiscriminate attachment;

- Exaggerated fearfulness;

- Depressed, withdrawn, apathetic;

- Sleep, speech or eating disorders;

- Substance abuse;

- Antisocial, destructive behaviour;

- Habit disorders (biting, rocking, whining, picking at scabs).

The Effects on Children Who Witness Family Violence:

Children who live in abusive homes may believe that they are responsible for the abuse. They learn early that violence is a way to solve problems and that people who hurt others are not being held accountable for this behaviour.

Some children may feel that they are the only ones who can stop the abuse, and this jeopardizes their safety.

Children in this environment also learn that inequality in relationships is normal and that men have power over women. They may believe that their mother deserves to be abused because of her weaknesses and they may then take on the role of the abuser because of this belief.

They may also believe that no matter what happens, there is no one to protect them. Therefore, their sense of trust in authority figures, such as police, teachers, counselors etc. is greatly diminished.

Chapter Seven

Eating Disorders

Anorexia Nervosa

- Refusal to maintain body weight at or above minimally normal weight for age and height (e.g. weight loss leading to maintenance of body weight less than 85% of that expected; or failure to make expected weight gain during period of growth, leading to body weight less than 85% of that expected).

- Intense fear of gaining weight or becoming fat, even though underweight.

- Disturbance in the way in which one's body weight or shape is experienced, undue influence of body weight or shape on self-evaluation, or denial of the seriousness of the current low body weight.

Specific types:

- **Restricting type:** During the episode of Anorexia Nervosa, the person has not regularly engaged in binge-eating or purging behaviour (i.e. self-induced vomiting or the misuse of laxatives, diuretics or enemas).

- **Binge-eating/purging type:** The person has regularly engaged in binge-eating or purging behaviour (i.e. self-induced vomiting or the misuse of laxatives, diuretics or enemas).

Associated features:

- Depressed mood;

- Somatic/sexual dysfunction;

- Guilt/obsession;

- Anxious/fearful/dependent personality of slenderness.

The Cycle of Bulimia Nervosa

- Fashion of slenderness;

- Self-dissatisfaction;

- Dieting;

- Weight loss;

- Disturbed sensation of hunger;

- Fasting;

- Vomiting, fear of becoming "fat" by overeating;

- Purging;

- Guilt, shame, disgust.

Bulimia Nervosa Medical Complications

- Bingeing;

- Acute stomach dilation;

- Risk of stomach rupture;

- Menstrual disorder (irregular or absent);

- Painless swelling of salivary glands;

- Vomiting;

- Dental decay (enamel injury);

- Chronic hoarseness and sore throat;

- Gastrointestinal reflex;

- Vomiting and laxative abuse;

- Metabolic disorders;

- Heart rhythm disorders;

- Dehydration

- Renal damage.

Diagnostic Criteria

- Repeated episodes of rapid consumption of large amounts of food (binge eating).

- A feeling of loss of control over eating behaviour during binge eating.

- In order to prevent weight gain, they regularly engage in self-induced vomiting, strict dieting or fasting, the use of laxatives or diuretics, or vigorous physical exercise.

- A minimum of two binge eating episodes per week for at least three months.

- Persistent preoccupation with the body and weight.

The Addiction Model

- Bulimia or excessive intake of food, especially sweet, rich food, can be considered a form of addiction.

- Various impulse control disorders and abuse of alcohol or drugs are observed in a good many of bulimia nervosa patients.

- Addictions in relatives of bulimia nervosa patients occur more frequently than in the normal population.

- The personality profile of bulimia nervosa patients shows strong similarities to that of alcoholics or drug addicts.

- Bulimia nervosa corresponds to the following criteria for addictions: loss of control, preoccupation with the substance, use of the substance to be able to deal with stress and negative feelings concealment, and persistence of addiction in spite of the repugnant results.

- The sociocultural context has a harmful impact on the family (from economic and political, as well as juridical points of view) and often results in the phenomenon of the "overprotecting" mother and the "absent" father.

- Most family problems are connected with problems about power and exceeding of boundaries in which men have greater social, economic, physical and political power than women.

- Many bulimics are victims of physical and sexual violence by men.

Why the Struggle Happens

Eating disorders are the result of a complex web of factors that include at least the following:

Stressful Situations

Emotional events in which teens do not possess coping skills usually lead to stress. Such situations may be rejection, a sexual encounter, or any number of other events. The peak age of onset for Anorexia coincides with the transition from junior high to high school. Bulimia most often occurs during the transition from high school to college.

Developmental Change

Adolescence is a period of great vulnerability to all kinds of struggles. For this reason, eating disorders are often seen as reactions to the stresses of puberty. Intimacy issues and responsibility may be avoided to some degree through maintenance of an eating disorder. Anorexics are characterized by extraordinary skill at following clear-cut rules. They are model children who have mastered good behaviour. Pre-anorexics are almost "too good to be true".

Biology

It is unclear whether an eating disorder produces the physiological changes or vice versa. Some researchers suggest that women may be biologically susceptible to eating disorders since they are far more likely than males to experience appetite fluctuation in response to stress.

Society

Two potential societal influences affect the increasing incidence of eating disorders. The first is the heightened consciousness of nutrition and physical fitness. In the last 2 to 3 decades, health and fitness have become major concerns. The second factor is our national obsession with slimness. In fact, we are willing to compromise the first factor, health, to achieve slimness.

Family Issues

Many agree that the family plays a leading role in the etiology of eating disorders—especially anorexia. Anorexic adolescents tend to come from families concerned about food. Mothers of adolescents who struggle with eating disorders may frequently have episodes of depression. Fathers are described as aloof or passive, yet with high expectations. However, no single set of parental personality traits have definitely been shown to exist universally.

Peer Relationships

During adolescence, peer groups are vital in easing the transition from childhood to adulthood. An absence of a group of friends is considered to be one feature in the onset of an eating disorder. Anorexics have a pattern of developing only one relationship at a time, and those relationships are repeatedly short-lived. They cheat themselves out of the aid of peers to help them through the process of individualization.

Anorexia:

- Voluntary starvation often leading to emaciation and sometimes death;

- Occasional binges, followed by fasting, laxative abuse, or self-induced starvation;

- Menstrual period ceases;

- Menstrual period may not begin if anorexia occurs before puberty;

- Excessive exercise;

- Hands, feet, and other parts of the body are always cold;

- Dry skin;

- Head hair may thin out;

- Fuzz may appear on other parts of the body;

- Depression;

- Irritability;

- Deceitfulness;

- Guilt;

- Self-loathing.

Bulimia

This action is best described as secretive binge eating. This can occur regularly and may follow a pattern. Caloric intake per binge can range from 100 to 20,000 calories.

Binges are followed by fasting, laxative abuse, self-induced vomiting, or other forms of purging. Person may chew food but spit it out before swallowing.

- Menstrual period may be regular, irregular or absent;

- Swollen glands in neck beneath jaw;

- Dental cavities and loss of tooth enamel;

- Broken blood vessels in face. Bags under eyes.

- Fainting spells. Rapid or irregular heartbeat.

- Miscellaneous stomach and intestinal discomforts and problems;

- Weight fluctuation due to alternating periods of binges and fasts;

- Desire for relationships and approval of others;

- Loses control and fears she cannot stop once she begins eating.

Chapter Eight

Sexual Activity

Many people decide to begin sexual activity for the wrong reasons: curiosity, they feel everyone else is doing it; they are trying to keep a boyfriend or girlfriend; they don't know what to say to a date; as women, they want to be "fulfilled"; and as males, they want to prove they are men.

Facts about teenage sexual activity:

- Within six months after becoming sexually active, half of all teenage girls become pregnant.

- Most teenagers do not use contraceptives until they have been sexually active for about nine months. Most just hope that they won't get pregnant.

- Eight out of ten pregnant teenagers drop out of school.

In fact, at least 50 percent of girls and 40 percent of boys are still virgins at their high school graduation. Don't let the bragging of others influence you or make you feel out of it.

Don't be deceived when you are watching music videos or reading celebrity magazines, because they can confuse you and make you feel that everyone spends their entire life partying.

Pros and Cons of Teenage Sexual Activity:

Negative Effects:

- Unwanted pregnancy;

- STD (sexually transmitted diseases);

- Requires lots of decisions: birth control methods, how to deal with your parents;

- Decrease in casual, friendly dating and an emphasis is placed on sex during dating;

- Feeling of being used after break-up.

Positive Effects:

- A way to try to "hold on to" a boyfriend or girlfriend;

- Feeling of being loved;

- Feeling older, more mature.

Of course you want to keep your boyfriend or girlfriend and to feel loved. There are other ways to do this without being sexually active and risking the sometimes severe consequences of that activity.

Pregnancy is a risk if you are sexually involved. It can complicate not only your family's life, but also that of your partner, your partner's parents, and the life of the unborn child. You have your life ahead of you

There is no need to rush this decision or take risks.

You can avoid sexual activity by avoiding situations that will oĕer opportunity. For example, don't go to your friend's house when you know that there is no adult there; plan activities when you go out on a date instead of just driving around; date in groups; go to indoor theatres instead of drive-ins; and think of some interesting subjects to talk about ahead of time.

The safest way to avoid all of the risks is to not become sexually involved at all (abstinence).

HIV/AIDS

HIV stands for Human Immunodeficiency Virus, which is the virus that causes AIDS (Acquired Immunodeficiency Syndrome). The virus attacks the body's immune system, which is your defense against infections.

How HIV/AIDS is spread:

The virus is spread from an infected person to someone else when there is an exchange of body fluids such as blood, semen, or vaginal fluids. This can occur during sexual intercourse or when contaminated needles are shared. A pregnant woman can infect her baby at the time of birth, and afterward during breastfeeding. Pregnant women should ask for an HIV test. HIV is not spread by everyday social contact. Touching, hugging and shaking hands with an infected person is safe. Insects and pets cannot spread HIV.

How to tell if you have HIV

A simple blood test can tell if you are infected with HIV. It is called the HIV antibody test. A positive test result means that you have been infected and that you can spread it to others. A negative result means that no antibodies to HIV were found in your blood at the time of testing.

Most positive tests will show up at three months, but HIV antibodies can take as long as six months to develop, so you need to get tested a second time to be certain you don't have the virus. AIDS is the last stage of HIV infection.

Infected people may get infections such as an unusual type of pneumonia, or develop skin cancer or other types of cancers.

How to lower the chances
of being infected with HIV:

- You can avoid HIV by not having sex at all, or by making sure that you protect yourself by always practicing "safe" sex with a partner who agrees to protect both of you by using a latex condom.

- Avoid using any instruments that pierce the skin unless you are sure they have been sterilized.

- Do not share personal items such as razors and toothbrushes.

If you think you may be infected:

If you have taken chances and are worried that you might be infected with HIV, see your doctor right away, or go to an HIV testing clinic or STD clinic. The blood test for HIV will be done, and all information will be kept private.

If you have been exposed to HIV, then your sex partners, or anyone with whom you have shared needles and syringes, must be told that they also may have been exposed to the virus. They will have to decide if they wish to be tested for HIV infection.

How HIV/AIDS is treated:

There is no cure for HIV infection or for AIDS at this time. The virus remains in the body for life. Several drugs have been developed recently that may slow the process of HIV but so far, none of them is a cure. However, a great deal of progress has been made and work is still continuing.

Children and HIV/AIDS

Children are vulnerable to infection through mother to child transmission during pregnancy or during birth. HIV can also be transmitted through breast milk. In Canada, 71% of HIV positive children were infected from their mothers, while the remaining were infected through transfusions of blood and blood products.

Children who are at high risk include those who are victims of sexual abuse, children in the sex trade, refugee and displaced children, and children in detention. Youth who become sexually active at an early age and those involved in injection drug use are also at a greater risk for HIV infection.

Children are not only infected by HIV, they are also affected. While the number of those infected by HIV continues to grow, the epidemic is also having a direct and devastating effect on millions of other children whose lives have been permanently altered by the intrusion of HIV/AIDS into their households or communities.

Children living in hard-hit communities feel the impact as they lose parents, teachers, and caregivers to AIDS, as health systems are stretched beyond their limits, and as their families take in other children who have been orphaned by the epidemic. The World Health Organization estimates that more than 3,000,000 children have been infected with HIV since the onset of the epidemic. It has been predicted that this number would continue to increase dramatically.

Children who are at increased risk of HIV infection include girls sought by men as sex partners on the belief that they are "safe"; street children who are vulnerable to sexual exploitation and who are often uneducated about risk behaviour; children who experience sexual abuse; and those who become sexually active at an early age.

What You Need to Know about
Sexually Transmitted Diseases (STD)

A teenager is nine times more likely to get an STD than an adult. Some people with an STD have few or no symptoms at all; others have very obvious symptoms.

Be aware of any changes in your health, or symptoms such as:

- Different or heavier discharge from the vagina;

- Discharge from the penis;

- A burning feeling when urinating;

- Sores, particularly in the genital or anal areas;

- Itching feeling around the sex organs or anus;

- Appearance of rash;

- Swollen glands in the groin.

These symptoms might appear alone, or in combinations.

What are your chances of catching an STD?

You have a chance of catching a sexually transmitted disease if:

- You have unprotected sex (without using a latex condom or if the condom breaks) with a person who may have an infection;

- You have a new partner;

- Your partner has sex with others;

- You are a user of injection drugs, or your partner is;

- You share needles for drugs, body piercing or tattoos, or your partner does.

Types of STD's

Chlamydia (pronounced kla-mid-ee-ah)

A very common sexually transmitted disease, this is one of the more serious. It can spread silently in the female and cause a painful, long-term condition called PID (Pelvic Inflammatory

Disease) and infertility. Pregnant women can pass this infection on to their babies, who can then get infections in their eyes or lungs.

You can get Chlamydia from vaginal or oral sex.

A young woman may never know she is infected with Chlamydia until she has a test for it or decides to have a baby and has problems trying to become pregnant.

For those who develop symptoms, these usually appear one to three weeks after sex with an infected person. Sometimes the symptoms are so mild that a person may not notice them. Men sometimes have no symptoms and can spread it without knowing they have it. It is very important that Chlamydia be treated immediately after detection.

What to look for:

Females

- A new or different discharge from the vagina;

- A burning feeling when urinating;

- A pain in the lower abdomen, sometimes with fever and chill;

- Pain during sex;

- Bleeding after intercourse.

Males

- A watery or milky drip from the penis;

- An itchy feeling inside the penis;

- A burning feeling when urinating;

- Pain or swelling in the testicles.

How Chlamydia is treated:

Chlamydia is treated with antibiotics taken orally.

Gonorrhea

You may hear of this STD by other names such as "the clap" or "a dose". Gonorrhea is a common STD, which if not treated early can cause serious health problems, especially for women.

- A pregnant woman can pass gonorrhea to her baby during birth, and cause a serious eye infection or blindness;

- You can get gonorrhea from oral, vaginal and anal sex;

- If you contract gonorrhea from having sex with an infected partner, you might not notice any symptoms. If you do, they will appear three to five days after sex.

What to look for:

Females

- New or different discharge from the vagina;

- A burning feeling when urinating;

- Pain in the lower abdomen;

- Fever and chills;

- Pain during sex.

Males

- Burning feeling when urinating;

- Pain or swelling in the testicles;

- Discharge from the penis, may be thick and yellow-green in colour.

How gonorrhea is treated:

Gonorrhea is treated with antibiotics and can be cured. But you can get it again right away from your partner if he/she has it and isn't getting treated as well.

Yeast infections

Normally, the vagina keeps itself healthy but sometimes too much yeast will grow in it, and cause a problem. Using birth control pills, taking antibiotics and sometimes certain foods, or hormone changes such as pregnancy, may cause yeast to grow.

If you have sex when you have a yeast infection, chances are your partner will not get it. But some men may find their penis gets red and itchy afterward.

There are medicines in the drugstore to treat yeast infections, but it is best to let a doctor diagnose the infection.

Genital Herpes

Herpes is an STD that causes painful sores on or around the genitals. Genital herpes is spread by direct contact with open sores, usually during sex. If you touch herpes sores, wash your hands with soap and water to avoid spreading the disease.

You can get genital herpes through oral sex—and even from cold sores. After the sores from the first attack heal, the herpes sores may appear from time to time.

There is no cure for genital herpes, but medication may shorten the attacks and make the sore less painful.

The symptoms and signs:

- Tingling or itching in the genital area may appear within a week of having sex with an infected person.

- A cluster of tiny blisters appear. These blisters burst and leave painful sores, which last from two to three weeks.

- A fever and headache may occur during the first attack.

What to look for:

Females

- Sores inside or near the vagina, on the genitals, near the anus, or on the thighs and buttocks;

- Tender lumps in the groin.

Males

- Sores in the penis, around the testicles, near the anus, and on the thighs and buttocks;

- Tender lumps in the groin.

Both males and females can get sores in the mouth or in the genital area after oral sex with an infected person.

Keep the infected area clean and dry. Wash your towel before re-using. After bathing, use a hair dryer instead of a towel around the sores, or gently pat dry.

Hepatitis B

This is an infection of the liver caused by a virus. It is much easier to get than HIV (AIDS).

Hepatitis B cannot be cured. Sometimes the infection goes away by itself, and sometimes people carry the virus for the rest of their lives and never know it.

It is the only sexually transmitted disease that can be prevented by a vaccine.

Most people who become infected with Hepatitis B have no symptoms.

Symptoms usually occur within two or six months after contact. They can include:

- Poor appetite, nausea and vomiting;

- Headaches;

- Feeling very tired;

- A general feeling of being unwell;

- Jaundice (yellow colouring of the eyes and skin).

How Hepatitis B is spread:

The Hepatitis B virus is spread through infected body fluids such as blood, semen and vaginal fluid.

If you are having sex (or if your regular sex partner has Hepatitis B), get a Hepatitis B vaccine from the doctor or public health clinic.

Hepatitis B is NOT ALWAYS an STD. You can get it other ways as well, so it is always a good idea to check with your doctor before you go on a vacation.

The Root of the Problem

In the animal kingdom it is survival of the fittest. Mankind is better than that, or are we?

Bullies are predators. And like any predatory animal the bully attacks those they consider weak, maimed or any other way inferior. Their arrogance puts them beyond fear of recrimination for their actions, in their mind everyone is afraid of them.

You can't reason with a bully, any attempt to do so is just another sign of weakness.

Our history books are full of war after war after war. And what is war if not the ultimate act of bullying? And this might is right mentality has become the driving force behind almost all aspects of our life.

In politics, attack ads and smear campaigns have taken priority over who can do a better job if elected.

In the corporate world, bigger is better. Hostile takeovers are considered signs of strength and power.

In sports, boxing, wrestling and ultimate fighting are a constant fixture on TV. Hockey has become a haven for bullies where superstars are targeted for career-ending head shots because of hard plastic elbow pads designed to afford maximum protection to the aggressor. Professional football had a scandal where a bounty was placed on opposing players. In baseball, a pitcher will throw a 100 mph fastball at a batter for crowding the plate of for hitting a homerun at the previous at bat. In soccer, player fall like bowling pins. Intimidation and physical superiority are what our children are led to believe is the best way to become rich, famous and respected.

Video games for children feature hard-core violence and killing with a laughable warning that the games are designed for a mature youth market.

And now we want to know why we have so many bullies in our schools.

Who has the answer?

For every sensationalized problem there are many so-called experts and solutions. Those in the medical profession want to find a treatable cause for the bully's behaviour. In the field of education, they believe society must have

(Continued from back cover)

made them that way, we should determine what we did wrong. The media find it more noteworthy (and a lot easier) to sensationalize the victim's background and blame them for what happened.

Zero tolerance (where any and all physical contact is punished) is not the solution. To the bully it is just a challenge to pick another time, another place. In fact, that policy only hinders the victim's first line of defense. If no witnesses step forward (and they rarely do) then who can tell who is lying about the alleged incident? How can the principal of a school be expected to determine who the real victim is?

The victim is the only true expert and all too often no one is hearing their cries for help. Imagine how they must feel when others stand by and watch, afraid to intervene lest they become the next target.

Why You Should Read This Book

In *The Death of Bullying*, we show you how to eliminate bullying from your child's school environment. It will take time, it will take social interaction, **it will save lives**. Parents owe it to their children, schools owe it to their students, School Boards owe it to their principals and teachers. They all want to see bullying stopped and now there are no more excuses for not putting an end to this social evil.

It is too late to help those unfortunate teens who have or are still committing suicide while we are standing helplessly on the sidelines. Can you say you don't have time, let someone else do it, it's not my child (can you really be so certain), and still look at yourself in the mirror?

About the Authors:

Dale Hirons: Has been involved in community activities for the past 25 years. Dale operated a youth centre for 15 years, sat on the Bridgeburg Neighbourhood Plan, obtained a grant from the Federal Government National Crime Prevention Program, and wrote a report on Revitalizing Our Neighbourhoods. While President of the Rose Seaton Public School PTA, he started a school breakfast program. Dale contributed to two Brock University studies: one by Dr. Heather Lee Kilty on Health and Wellness Fort Erie, and one by Dr. Hans Skott-Myrhe, Dr. Rebecca Raby and Jamie Nikolau on Fort Erie Youth Living Without Secure Housing.

After 12 years of research, Dale began to put the information he was compiling on paper. His years of fact-finding are the backbone of this Anti-Bullying Policy, a one-of-a-kind approach that is proactive rather than reactive, which is the model most other programs are based on.

Robert Hirons: As a long-time supervisor in the workplace Robert has seen the best and worst of behaviour as company employees tried to improve their status. When he became a foreman, his found out his supervisor operated under the assumption that the best way to achieve the desired results was to be a bully. The foremen in his department had to work under these conditions or lose their jobs.

His son also experienced bullying first-hand. At school he was a target of bullies because of his size. He didn't want his father to think he was a sissy, so he never mentioned it at home. At that time, (much like too many schools today) there was no policy in place at school to deal with the problems he faced on a daily basis. Robert was never told this until they discussed the book Dale was working on, and that was when Robert became involved in the project.

Gary Hirons: In school, Gary's shyness made him an outsider. He never got to participate in many of the extra-curricular activities because of his inability to make friends. He felt he was alone, even when trying to participate in group activities.

As an older member of a large family Gary has been a helpful uncle to several nieces and nephews. He has coached some of them in baseball and hockey and could readily tell which opposing coaches were more concerned with winning than skill development. Those young children responded best to authority, respect, friendship and fairness.

For the past year he has been working with Dale on this project.

Writing This Book

When we began to study the effects of bullying on students, we had no idea of the scope of information on available on the subject. After a great deal of research and reading, we realized that the "experts" were all reactive, trying to work with the bullies to teach them the error of their ways. We believe the only way to truly and effectively eliminate bullying is to use a proactive approach. Only then will our children be safe at school. This book educates teachers, parents and students on how to ensure their school will have a learning environment safe from fear.